Hays cuts through theoretical jargon like butter and translates it into practical wisdom that readers can use to directly improve their lives. I'm thrilled to have this book to recommend to clients, and as a person on the journey through a stress-filled life, I'm pleased to have it guide me toward a greater sense of positive, strength-based well-being.

—John Sommers-Flanagan, PhD, *Professor of Counselor Education, College of Education and Human Sciences, University of Montana, Missoula*

Most people are searching for something more out of life. Hays teaches us how to find it. She makes well-being a realistic goal for us all.

—Shane J. Lopez, PhD, *Research Director, Clifton Strengths Institute, Omaha, NE*

Hays has brilliantly condensed decades of psychological science into an easy-to-read manual for creating a life of happiness and fulfillment.

—Brad Klontz, PhD, *Financial Psychologist, Associate Professor, Kansas State University, Manhattan; author of* Mind Over Money: Overcoming the Money Disorders That Threaten Our Financial Health

Packed with excellent research-based strategies, this book is an invaluable source for anyone interested in living well. Highly recommended!

—Lillian Comas-Díaz, PhD, *Clinical Professor, The George Washington University, Department of Psychiatry and Behavioral Sciences, Washington, DC; author of* Multicultural Care: A Clinician's Guide to Cultural Competence

Creating
Well-Being

Creating Well-Being

FOUR STEPS TO A HAPPIER, HEALTHIER LIFE

PAMELA A. HAYS, PhD

American Psychological Association • Washington, DC

Published by
American Psychological Association
750 First Street, NE
Washington, DC 20002
www.apa.org

To order
APA Order Department
P.O. Box 92984
Washington, DC 20090-2984
Tel: (800) 374-2721;
Direct: (202) 336-5510
Fax: (202) 336-5502;
TDD/TTY: (202) 336-6123
Online: www.apa.org/books/
E-mail: order@apa.org

In the U.K., Europe, Africa, and the Middle East, copies may be ordered from
American Psychological Association
3 Henrietta Street
Covent Garden, London
WC2E 8LU England

Typeset in Sabon by Circle Graphics, Columbia, MD

Printer: Edwards Brothers, Lillington, NC
Cover Designer: Naylor Design, Washington, DC

The opinions and statements published are the responsibility of the authors, and such opinions and statements do not necessarily represent the policies of the American Psychological Association.

Library of Congress Cataloging-in-Publication Data
Hays, Pamela A.
    Creating well-being : four steps to a happier, healthier life / Pamela A. Hays.
        pages cm
    Includes bibliographical references and index.
    ISBN-13: 978-1-4338-1573-7
    ISBN-10: 1-4338-1573-7
    1. Happiness. 2. Well-being. I. Title.
    BF575.H27H394 2014
    152.4'2—dc23
                                            2013018096

British Library Cataloguing-in-Publication Data
A CIP record is available from the British Library.

Printed in the United States of America
First Edition

http://dx.doi.org/10.1037/14317-000

CONTENTS

Contents

ACKNOWLEDGMENTS

I would like to thank Marjorie and Hugh Hays for their helpful suggestions and unwavering support. I am grateful to Mary Ann Boyle and Paul Landen for their feedback on an initial draft, to Tim Gillis for sharing his idea of the thought train, and to Kelsi Staton for permission to use her drawing of the thought train. I also want to thank Maureen Adams for supporting this project and Tyler Aune for his helpful ideas and excellent editing. Finally, I am deeply grateful to my husband, Bob McCard, for his proofreading, suggestions, encouragement, and support.

Creating
Well-Being

INTRODUCTION

Marisol works full-time in a busy hospital, coaches a girls' soccer team, and raises two teenagers with her partner who also works full time.[1] Marisol describes herself as "majorly stressed out" and acknowledges her perfectionist tendencies. She says she worries about everything—most recently, their debt and the kids' upcoming college expenses. She has trouble sleeping, feels anxious a lot, and has gained weight from overeating. Sometimes she feels trapped and despairs that she will ever feel any peace.

Sheldon is a single young manager for a company that has high expectations of its employees. His live-in girlfriend moved out 3 months ago because, as she told him, she was "tired of always being second" after his work. Sheldon has been drinking more than he knows he should, finds it difficult to get out of bed in the morning, and has been irritable with his coworkers. He knows what he wants in life—a family, a comfortable home, and more fun—but feels deeply discouraged about the likelihood that he will ever have these things.

Carol is in her 60s, and after raising three children and caring for her mother-in-law, she has returned to working full-time and loves it. However, her retired husband is pressuring her to quit and

---

[1]Unless noted otherwise, the people described in this book are composites and not representative of any single individuals.

stay home, their grown daughter wants her to babysit the grandkids, and the church wants her to resume her volunteer activities. Carol feels a mixture of guilt, frustration, and anger, which she ignores until someone triggers her anger and she yells at them, which makes her feel even guiltier.

Despite their differences, Marisol, Sheldon, and Carol have one thing in common: All are experiencing painful emotions and engaging in behaviors that add to their stress. Marisol tries to fix everything and help everyone, then eats to calm herself when she can't do it all. Sheldon snaps at coworkers, withdraws from family and friends, then drinks to feel better. Carol tries to be "nice" by holding in her frustration until she can't anymore, then blows up at whomever is there, increasing her feelings of guilt, which leads her to try even harder to hold it all in. All three have tried everything they know to feel better and do better, but even when they make a change, it doesn't last and they wind up feeling worse.

Perhaps you find yourself in a similar situation—stressed out, overwhelmed, repeating behaviors that work against you. Would you like to have more control over your emotions, to act in ways that fit with your values and who you want to be? Do you want to be physically and mentally healthier, and to have healthier relationships? Do you wish you could enjoy your life more, that happiness and well-being could be your norm?

If you answered yes to any of these questions, this book is for you. *Creating Well-Being: Four Steps to a Happier, Healthier Life* will help you build your personal well-being, which in turn will positively affect the well-being of others. With this user-friendly toolbox of exercises, tips, and strategies, you will learn how to do the following:

- recognize and use your personal strengths to maximum effect;
- solve problems with confidence and calm;

- manage difficult emotions in the face of problems you cannot control;
- build healthy, mutually satisfying relationships; and
- appreciate what you have and enjoy life more.

THE TOOLBOX

During my 20-plus years as a psychologist, I have studied many different approaches to living well, and this book contains the best of everything I have learned and found to work. I use these tools in my life every day, I teach them to clients in my clinical practice and to student psychologists and counselors, and I share them with my family and friends.

The toolbox consists of my own combination of the most effective, easy-to-understand practices from three influential areas of psychology. The first area, known as *positive psychology,* turns traditional psychology on its head by shifting the focus from individual problems and weaknesses to human strengths and potential. Positive psychology is primarily a research-oriented field that includes a wealth of studies pinpointing the elements of and contributors to happiness and well-being, including the role of relationships, meaning, and purpose. Positive psychologists seek to understand kindness; generosity; humor; optimism; courage; hope; and other positive qualities, experiences, and conditions that play a part in the well-being of individuals, communities, and nations. Some of their findings contradict long-held beliefs about what makes people happy—information that I include in this book.

The second area I draw from is the most widely used form of psychotherapy, *cognitive–behavioral therapy,* or CBT. If you think of positive psychology as a pair of glasses you put on to see the strengths and positive possibilities in yourself and others, CBT is the set of tools for building these strengths in yourself, growing into your potential, and positively affecting others. These tools have been used by psychotherapists for decades to help people manage emotions, change behavior, decrease stress, improve relationships, and get healthy.

CBT's basic premise is that what we *think* affects how we *feel,* which in turn affects what we *do.* It is a mind–body approach that also includes strategies for listening to your body's cues regarding what you need and taking action to change your behavior or situation in ways that build emotional, physical, and social well-being. CBT is not just about thinking positively or a Polyanna-ish smear of happy thoughts replacing problems. Rather, it is about thinking more *realistically* by looking for and recognizing positive possibilities in the face of problems, because when we are stressed, we tend to overlook the positives and focus on the negatives, which then aggravates the problem and our stress.

CBT focuses on the creation of healthy, desired *change* (even when the change is only in one's thinking), but sometimes change is impossible or extremely difficult (including changing one's thinking). This is where the third influential area of *mindfulness* comes in.

Mindfulness refers to a state of mind involving moment-to-moment awareness without judgment of anything or anyone. *Mindfulness practices,* such as meditation, work in part by decreasing the emotional reactivity that magnifies emotional upset and physical pain. This decreased reactivity makes acceptance of yourself and what's going on around you easier, which is especially important when you have no control over events anyway. Mindfulness practices aid in building awareness and acceptance of internal experience (thoughts, feelings, physical sensations) and external events that you cannot change. It is also used to build a compassionate and patient attitude that facilitates action. In summary, positive psychology describes the elements of well-being, CBT provides the tools to build it, and mindfulness increases those tools' effectiveness.

Marisol, Sheldon, and Carol are each facing stressful life events, but each is also engaging in particular ways of thinking and behaviors that add to their stress. Marisol holds perfection as the gold standard for her life and behavior, and when she does not meet it, she berates herself, which leads her to feel worse and then overeat, which fuels her harsh self-talk even further. Sheldon goes over and over in his mind his dissatisfaction with himself and others, how hard he works, the unfairness of his girlfriend—thoughts that increase his anger and lead him to drink and treat others harshly, damaging the other relationships he still has. Carol holds an unspoken belief that works against her well-being: the belief that a good person is someone who always puts others first. This belief leads her to ignore her own needs and desires until they build to the point at which she explodes emotionally, which then fuels her belief that she is not a good person and needs to try harder by ignoring her own needs even more.

As you will see in subsequent chapters, with the help of the thought-change tools, Marisol, Sheldon, and Carol learn to recognize and then change their harmful thinking patterns, thoughts, beliefs, and images to ones that build their well-being. These changes in thinking then help them take positive actions, including changing their situations and behavior, in ways that further build their well-being.

USING THIS BOOK

Imagine well-being as a path and this book as a supportive companion on your path. If you are experiencing mild to moderate anxiety, depression, anger, fear, jealousy, or other unwanted emotions, or engaging in repetitive self-defeating behaviors, this book will help you decrease those unwanted emotions, eliminate stressors when possible, and engage in thinking and behaviors that build your well-being.

These tools can also be obtained through psychotherapy, but I have found that most people prefer to try changing on their own first. So to make this easy to do, I have written the book in a self-help format that you can use by yourself. But keep in mind that if you decide to find a psychotherapist, the book can be used in conjunction with therapy too. Therapists may find the book helpful as a guide in their work with clients, particularly because it provides a step-by-step approach with practice exercises.

Please be advised that for some people, this book will probably not be enough. Trying to deal with severe depression or anxiety on your own is not advised. If you are experiencing severe symptoms that significantly impair your daily functioning, I strongly recommend that you find a good therapist. Severe emotional symptoms can skew your thinking to the point that it becomes extremely difficult to change on your own. For example, if you feel trapped and truly believe that you have no options, a therapist can perceive possibilities that you don't and help you minimize your pain and change behaviors that worsen the situation or your stress. You can certainly still make use of this book, but a skilled therapist can help you tailor the tools to your specific needs.

I have organized the book's contents according to the four main steps I undertake with clients in my clinical practice. These are:

- Step 1: *Stepping Onto the Path of Well-Being,*
- Step 2: *Understanding Your Stressors,*
- Step 3: *Using Thoughts to Feel Better,* and
- Step 4: *Taking Action.*

Because most people are pretty discouraged by the time they seek help, Step 1: *Stepping Onto the Path of Well-Being,* provides inspiration and encouragement. *Inspiration* is related to the word *respiration* and literally means to *breathe life into*, whereas *encouragement* comes from the word *courage*. I emphasize both inspiration and encouragement because I have found that even when one feels full of life and ready to go, change still takes courage. To inspire and encourage you, Step 1 includes exercises that will help you imagine what well-being looks like for *you*, clarify the values you consider important to who you are and who you want to be, and recognize what you already have going for you.

Step 2: *Understanding Your Stressors*, teaches you to recognize stress that is *internally generated* by thoughts, beliefs, and interpretations and to distinguish it from stress that is *externally generated* by situations and other people. Stress from both sources diminishes a person's well-being, but recognizing the source helps in deciding which tools to use to address the problem. Because the body is a treasure chest of information regarding the effects of stress and well-being, this step includes mindfulness practices that will help you tap into your body's messages regarding your needs and what might help to meet them. These messages will enable you to recognize stressors that you may not previously have recognized as such and to understand their unique psychological and physical effects on you.

Steps 3 and 4 involve learning and using the two main types of tools I describe in this book: thought-change tools and action tools. Step 3, *Using Thoughts to Feel Better*, provides thought-change tools that build well-being by changing negatively skewed thoughts, thinking patterns, and beliefs to more realistic ones that recognize and maximize the positive. You will learn how to avoid thought traps that block your path and replace harsh, judgmental self-talk with a compassionate voice that facilitates personal growth and relationships. You will also learn how to shape your self-talk in ways that increase your acceptance of problems that you cannot directly change (such as other people's behavior or a medical problem) and take action to change problems that you *can* change (such as situational factors and your own behavior).

Step 4, *Taking Action,* focuses on action tools for changing your behavior or your environment. To help you remember all of the action tools, I have organized them into five categories, which I call the *CLASS* actions:

- Create a healthy environment;
- Learn and practice well-being behavior;
- Assertiveness, conflict resolution, and other communication skills;
- Social engagement, meaning, and purpose; and
- Self-care for staying on the happy, healthy path.

Within each of these categories, I describe specific tools for building your well-being.

For the purposes of this book, I have put the thought-change tools before the action tools, but you may decide that starting with the action tools works better for you in a given situation, and that is fine. Changing unhelpful thinking often makes it easier to take action, but sometimes small, easy action steps make you feel so much better that the negative thoughts and feelings are no longer a problem.

For example, if you are experiencing a great deal of loneliness and an easy first step for you involves attending a group you know you enjoy, then by all means go to the group. Because it is a group you enjoy, the experience is likely to build positive emotions and thoughts, making it easier for you to take further action to decrease your loneliness. However, if you believe that most people don't like you and won't welcome you, a better first step might be to work on changing your belief to a more realistic, helpful one that will make the action step easier and increase the likelihood that you will experience positive interactions when you are ready to reach out. In my clinical practice, I usually ask people which they think would be the easiest place to start: changing unhelpful thinking or taking small action steps. I encourage individuals to use *the path of least resistance principle* to decide—that is, to choose the easiest approach because change is already difficult enough.

Throughout the book, I include exercises for thinking about and trying these new ideas, tips, and strategies. In addition, at the end of every chapter, there is a Small Step exercise that encourages you to practice something new for at least 1 week. In my clinical practice, this Small Step is the homework I give clients between therapy sessions, which typically occur once a week. For this reason, I would suggest reading only one chapter per week, to allow yourself time to think about the ideas in that chapter over a period of several days.

I emphasize moving forward with small steps for three reasons. One, small steps are easier to do, so they quickly create a feeling of success. Two, there is something energizing about taking a first step, even if it is small. And three, because small steps are easier to integrate into your busy life, you are more likely to stick with them.

This book is an interactive experience that involves effort and patience. Your thought patterns include deeply held beliefs that took a long time to develop, and it is highly unlikely that you will move overnight from the negative end of an emotion to its opposite (e.g., from rage to acceptance). To reap the maximum benefits, you will need to commit to your path of well-being and be patient with yourself. The steps and tools may feel a bit goofy at first, because new behavior always feels odd, but keep at it and watch the positive effects grow. The longer you practice the tools, the better they work. As you gradually change your thoughts and actions, your feelings will follow, and as you feel better, thought change will become easier in what I call the *positive snowball effect.*

Even in the most difficult times, each of us has an internal strength that acts as a compass, pointing us toward wellness. You are the expert on your life, so use these tools as they work best for you. My hope is that with this book you will gain a deeper understanding and appreciation of yourself and others and live a life that is full of purpose, meaning, and joy.

Step 1:

STEPPING ONTO THE PATH OF WELL-BEING

CHAPTER I

FINDING *YOUR* PATH

Step forward into your life as you did when you were a child,
when you believed anything was possible.

—Vince Gowman

Making changes in your life requires the belief that change will
lead to something better. Although you may not see all of the
positive possibilities now, clarifying your values, hopes, and
dreams can get you going in the direction you want to go, onto
the path of well-being.

I was visiting my friend Al in another state after a few years of not seeing him, and in the course of our talk, I asked him, "Are you happy?"
He looked surprised and said, "I don't really think about that," but
then proceeded to tell me how much he liked his new townhouse
and the neighbors he considered friends, how engaged he was with
his work as a teacher, and how much he enjoyed weekend trips with
his partner and playing with his beloved dog. His description of his
comfortable home, close community, meaningful work, love, and
fun sounded like more than happiness; it sounded like *well-being.*

Happiness is a word we use a lot in conversation, but its
meaning can be elusive, and it often means different things to different people. For this reason, psychologists tend to focus instead on
well-being, a broader concept that includes happiness and a whole
lot more. Well-being refers to the wellness of one's whole being—

emotional, cognitive, physical, social, and spiritual. And well-being is not just about *being* well yourself, it is also about *doing* well, that is, acting in ways that increase the well-being of others.

Although psychologists agree that having the basic needs of food and shelter met is a prerequisite for well-being, they differ in how they frame the elements of well-being. For the purposes of this book, I focus on four elements that most agree are key: happiness, mental and physical health, healthy relationships, and purpose. Let's take a moment to consider each of these.

ELEMENTS OF WELL-BEING

Happiness

Happiness consists of two inextricably linked components: positive emotions (the *feelings* part) and satisfaction with one's life (the *cognitive* part; Diener & Biswas, 2008). Because people who are highly satisfied with their lives feel good much of the time, positive emotion is core to what we think of as happiness and well-being.

Take a moment to think about your own happiness with the questions in the box below.

Try This

On a scale of 0 (*very negative*) to 10 (*very positive*), what level of positive emotion do you feel right now? _____
On a scale of 0 (*very unsatisfied*) to 10 (*very satisfied*), how satisfied are you with your life? _____

Are your two ratings similar? Do you see a connection between the two? Do you think your ratings might be different tomorrow, next week, or next year?

I have found it helpful to think of happiness as a by-product of the actions and ways of thinking that increase well-being. At times, these actions and thinking strategies may increase positive emotion without increasing life satisfaction. However, when enjoyable activities are devoid of meaning and purpose, they do not increase well-being.

This is not to say that play is useless. On the contrary, rest, leisure, and recreation are rejuvenating and necessary to keep us going; in this sense, they have a purpose. But perpetual pleasure seeking for its own sake leads to an emptiness that is the opposite of real happiness. Moreover, it is impossible to feel good constantly. Even if you have all the resources in the world and can schedule an unending series of enjoyable events, the human tendency to adapt means that you will continually need a bigger and better thrill to feel good. As we will see, happiness is linked to other aspects of well-being in interesting ways.

Mental and Physical Health

As Martin Seligman (one of the founders of positive psychology) pointed out, the problem with focusing solely on happiness as a measure of well-being is that too much emphasis is placed on a person's mood (Seligman, 2011). Happy emotions come and go, so there are times when you may not *feel* happy but still be satisfied with your life. Therefore, it is necessary to think about other measures of well-being that are just as important, such as mental and physical health.

Considering mental and physical health separately provides a fuller picture of well-being. For example, the psychological resilience that is a part of mental health enables a person to recognize problems and feel pain but, at the same time, to see helpful possibilities, engage with life, and experience positive emotions. Happy people are mentally healthy and vice versa. They are flexible and open to learning and growth.

Years ago, I worked in a variety of geriatric facilities and was impressed by the resilience of the older adults with whom I worked. These individuals usually had at least one medical condition in addition to one or more recent major life events, such as the death of a spouse or adult child or a move to an assisted-living facility with a subsequent cascade of losses. But even with such huge challenges and a diminished ability to physically meet these challenges, the people I met frequently surprised me with their sense of humor (a cognitive ability that brings with it positive emotion). Perhaps not surprisingly, studies now show that older people on average are happier than younger people (Haidt, 2006) and that longevity is linked to high levels of happiness (Diener & Chan, 2010). As my 80-year-old parents tell me, when you know you have fewer days left, you appreciate each one even more.

In addition to interactions with emotional and mental health, happiness and well-being positively affect physical health. Studies show that positive emotions and life satisfaction decrease the risk of heart problems, and more specifically, optimism decreases the risk of heart attack. A big part of this decreased risk relates to the greater social support that happier people experience. In a study conducted at the University of Rochester, happily married people who had heart bypass surgery were up to 3 times more likely to be alive 15 years later than their unmarried counterparts. For women, the effects were strongest when the marriage was a happy one, although for men, the support of any marriage was enough to increase longevity (King & Reis, 2012).

Healthy Relationships

Happiness is not a self-centered pursuit. In fact, personal happiness *increases* generosity, goodwill, and concern for others—a fact that is recognized by many different cultures. For example, the Inupiaq people of Alaska describe individual happiness with the term *aregah,* meaning *community well-being,* because in a small community in which everyone is related, the well-being of one affects the well-being of all. Similarly, Tibetan Buddhists believe that everything is interconnected, so caring for others is like caring for yourself. As the Dalai Lama (2009) has said, "If you want others to be happy, practice compassion. If *you* want to be happy, practice compassion" (p. 18).

Studies show that married people *are* happier. However, it is a chicken–egg question as to what causes what. Marriage *does* increase life satisfaction and opportunities for positive emotion, but it is also true that happiness increases the likelihood of marrying, because happy people are more attractive and easier to live with (Haidt, 2006). In any case, it is clear that healthy, mutually satisfying relationships are among the most powerful contributors to well-being. And in one of those wonderful paradoxes of life, the more you care for others, the more your own support grows.

Purpose

The life satisfaction component of well-being depends heavily on the meaning of one's choices and actions. A belief in something bigger than oneself has been clearly linked to happiness and well-being. More specifically, religious people report greater well-being than nonreligious people, partly because of the social support that comes with religious involvement but also because of the experience of transcendence and the sense of purpose that come with religious faith.

Of course, one does not have to be religious to have meaning, purpose, or even spirituality. For many people, meaning, purpose, and a sense of connectedness to something bigger than oneself come through helping others, working to improve the natural environment, joining a common cause, raising healthy children, and other such endeavors. I like to think of such beliefs as part of an internal compass that guides us toward our particular path of well-being, providing hope and a way to make it through the painful experiences that life brings.

FINDING YOUR PATH

In a workshop for psychotherapists that I once attended, psychologist Christine Padesky asked participants what they would say to a 7-year-old who says, "When I grow up, I want to be an astronaut!" The common response was something like, "Wow, that's great! What planet would you want to visit first?" But as Christine went on to say, if an adult in his or her late 40s tells you, "I've decided I want to be an astronaut," you'd probably say, "Hmmm. Isn't there an age limit on that?"

Although we encourage children to dream, when we become adults, we often stop dreaming. We set our sights on "realistic" goals and expect others to do the same. But realistic goals and big dreams are not incompatible. On the contrary, they can work together if your dreams inspire you to work toward your goals, and the goals steer you toward your dreams.

In thinking about how to create a path that will steer you toward your dreams, it is important to consider what you value. Human beings share many core values—for example, the desire for love, friendship, and fun. However, value *priorities* vary depending on one's upbringing, culture, and family. Even one's environment can affect one's values.

Being clear about your value priorities helps you imagine a path that fits who you are and who you want to be. The more details you imagine regarding your dream and the path toward that dream, the more able you will be to see the steps you need to take. Think of this as a three-part endeavor in which you (a) recognize your value priorities, (b) imagine living your dream in detail, and (c) imagine the steps you need to take on a path of well-being that fits with your values and takes you toward your dream.

When Marisol began thinking about what she values, she placed peace of mind at the top of her list. She realized that in her efforts to be more efficient and productive, she had let go of some of the activities that used to give her the experience of serenity. One of these activities was hiking. The stillness of the woods calmed her mind and body in a way that felt spiritual to her and carried over into the rest of her life, even when she was very busy. Another past activity was playing the piano, which took her outside herself. She also used to sketch, which involved focusing all of her attention in a way that was calming. Marisol began to imagine her life with these activities in it again and the peace they would bring. The more she thought about these activities as possibilities, the readier she felt to take a step toward this new path. Her first small step along these lines was the decision to set aside one Saturday or Sunday afternoon per month for a walk in the woods. She recognized that this would not change her life as much as she would like, but setting aside the time to begin building her well-being increased her hope that she could bring more peace into her life.

As Sheldon considered his value priorities, he realized that despite the high value he placed on having a family and a home, he had put his work first. However, he felt stuck because although he saw the need to build up his social life—especially now that he was single—he still felt pressured to work long hours, which kept him from socializing. Initially, he decided he would try organizing his office, because if he were more organized, he would work more efficiently and be able to leave work on time. But starting with a simple step such as sorting files was the opposite of inspiring—it was just one more thing he had to do, and having too much to do was part of his problem. So instead he began to think more about his dream of having a home, a wife, and kids, visualizing weekend barbecues with friends and family, being more fit from playing basketball (which he enjoyed but had quit doing), and feeling better because of eating healthier (which he rarely did because he didn't like cooking for himself). Picturing his dream life in detail helped him to see more inspiring small actions he could take to move himself toward an emotionally and physically healthier place. He decided to take one night per week to play basketball at the YMCA.

Carol was aware of the high value she placed on her relationships and helping others. She could not imagine her life without this as a central theme because it fit with her spiritual beliefs and gave her a sense of purpose. However, as Carol started dreaming about her own well-being, she began to see how her thinking, rather than the people around her, was the block to her well-being. She gradually began to change her definition of her personal needs as selfish by telling herself, "I was made this way for a reason, and just like I need to meet my physical needs for food, water, and sleep, paying attention to my emotional, social, and spiritual health will help me be a better human being."

The exercise in the box on the next page will help you think more about your values in relation to your life dreams and path. With your values front and center in your mind, now imagine your dream life. Where is it (geographically)? What is your home like? Who is around you, and what are your relationships like? What are you doing or not doing (e.g., fun activities, work, helping others, interests)? In this dream life, what have you accomplished or completed? What are you looking forward to? What are you grateful for?

Next, begin to connect this dream to the path that will take you there, keeping in mind the importance of small steps. As the examples of Marisol, Sheldon, and Carol illustrate, small steps will not solve your problems overnight. A small step may even seem futile in the face of everything that's going on. But consider this: When you're

Think About This: Values Priority List

Circle your top three values from the list below. If something that you value is missing, add and circle it.

1. Balance
2. Financial success
3. Fame
4. Love
5. Simplicity
6. Freedom
7. Spirituality
8. Gratitude
9. Courage
10. Nature/protecting the natural environment
11. Justice
12. Contributing to others
13. Power
14. Community
15. Creativity/self-expression
16. Physical fitness/health
17. Mental/emotional health
18. Other _____
19. Other _____
20. Other _____

Think about the ways in which your top three values influence your thinking, your behavior, your daily activities, and your relationships. Is your life currently in sync with these values? How or how not? _____

_____

driving in the dark at night with only your headlights illuminating the road, all you can see is what is right in front of you—but you can drive all the way from California to New York that way.

SMALL STEP

Continue to think about your dream life and the path of well-being that leads to it. If it helps, make a brief mental video of yourself moving along this path, keeping in mind that the path itself is one of greater happiness. Don't worry about taking any action steps at this point. For the next week, just replay your video once a day, and let your hopefulness grow.

CHAPTER 2

TAPPING YOUR HIDDEN STRENGTHS

There is in each of us so much goodness that if we could see it glow, it would light the world.

—Sam Friend

When you want to make a change, the first steps are usually the hardest, so it is important that they be easy to do. This chapter is aimed at inspiring you and encouraging you by focusing on everything you have going for you.

Most of us are painfully aware of our weaknesses and mistakes. Think about how many times in the past week you noted something you dislike about yourself—your weight, your hair, your difficulty with math, your shyness with new people, an error you made at work, whatever. Now think about how many times in the past week you noted something you *like* about yourself.

When we are stressed, any negative skew in our thoughts becomes even more pronounced. Psychologists call this tendency the *negative interpretation bias* because even positive events are interpreted negatively. For example, when a coworker told Sheldon he did an excellent job in coordinating a meeting, Sheldon thought to himself, "She's just trying to get in good with me because she wants something." This negative thought created a negative feeling (irritation), which led to a negative behavior (dismissal of the comment). Over time, Sheldon's negative attitude and behavior elicited irritation from his coworkers and anger from his partner, and their reactions made them feel worse about himself.

Like Sheldon, some people, when stressed, tend to externalize their frustration and blame others or events, whereas other people internalize their frustration and blame themselves for whatever happens. Studies show that women tend to internalize and men to externalize, but whatever your tendency, the result is the same: a negative bias that affects how you feel about yourself, the world around you, and the future.

But just as negativity snowballs, so too can positivity. Positive thinking creates and builds positive emotions, positive behaviors, and positive relationships. By studying the emotional lives of individuals and examining the data from research on couples and work teams, psychologist Barbara Fredrickson found what she called the *tipping point* at which thoughts and emotions snowball in one direction or the other (Fredrickson, 2012). When the ratio is at least three positive emotions to one negative emotion, positivity creates an energizing spiral up into even more positivity, creativity, and aliveness. Below this ratio, individuals and groups experience a negative spiral down that leads to persistent rigidity and lifelessness.

Fortunately, there are as many opportunities for positive thinking as there are for negative thinking, particularly when it comes to how you think about yourself. But because most of us are trained to be self-critical and the points of comparison around us are increasingly unrealistic (think fashion models, wealthy celebrities, "self-made" billionaires), shifting focus to your strengths requires some effort. In my clinical practice, one of the exercises I do to help people refocus is what I call a Personal Strengths Inventory (PSI). The PSI is a list of everything you have going for you.

If that nagging negative voice is kicking in right now with *Get real—I'll never be [fill in the blank] no matter how much I focus on my strengths; This is ridiculous;* or *I don't want to get carried away with myself—people will think I'm arrogant,* then keep the following in mind. I am not talking about making things up about yourself, for example, telling yourself you are the perfect weight if you are 50 pounds over what is healthy for you. What I *am* talking about is that even if you *are* 50 pounds overweight, consider shifting your focus to a more realistic one that recognizes all of the positive qualities, abilities, strengths, and supports you *do* have. This focus is not about ignoring something you want to change about yourself, it is about balancing your perspective to include the positive.

Shifting focus in this way can be hard, and in my clinical practice, I rarely ask people to do this on their own. Instead, I ask person-specific questions to help each individual recognize their strengths and supports. To help you with this, I've listed lots of examples below that you can choose from, but you may also want to ask for help from others. Think of a person or two who care about you and explain to them that you are trying to become more positive, starting with yourself. Ask if they would be willing to help you with appreciating everything you have going for you. In Sheldon's case, his mother and sister were delighted to give him positive input because they were tired of his irritability and negativity and wanted him to feel better.

Paying attention to your strengths and supports is a first step toward your path of well-being, and constructing your PSI is a concrete way to make this happen. Its purpose right now is to inspire and encourage you. But as you continue through this book, you will see how this positive focus on yourself will add to the other positive small steps you will take.

Before beginning your PSI, it is helpful to obtain a baseline of how you are feeling at present, so that later you can assess whether the exercise made a difference in how you feel. Rate your positive feeling right now on a scale of 0 (*feeling very negative, low, or lacking confidence*) to 10 (*feeling very positive, hopeful, and confident*). Write that number in the box on the next page.

<table>
</table>

Consider This

My Emotional Starting Point _____

CREATING YOUR PSI

The writing portion of this exercise is key for two reasons: (a) writing forces us to focus and think carefully (in this case, on the positives), and (b) at the end you will have a written record of your strengths and supports that will be needed in some of the strategies described later. So don't skip over the writing part by simply saying your strengths to yourself without writing them down. Also, to get the most out of this exercise, follow each step in order.

1. Circle all of the following positive qualities you recognize in yourself.

My Positive Qualities
I am:

kind	computer-	easy going	clean and
compassionate	savvy	sincere	sober
artistic	musical	courageous	open-minded
loyal	respectful	humble	trustworthy
independent	polite	helpful	capable
cooperative	committed	patient	dependable
persistent	bilingual	fair	healthy
intelligent	likeable	grateful	a survivor
creative	friendly	energetic	resourceful

trusting	strong	well-organized	physically
articulate	funny	stable	active
honest	a good listener	determined	skilled
attractive	attentive	curious	
hard working	outgoing	generous	

Now go to the page titled Personal Strengths Inventory on the last page of this chapter (p. 35). Under the section My Positive Qualities, write each of the qualities you circled, prefacing each with *I am* or *I have,* like this:

> *I am kind.*
> *I am compassionate.*
> *I have good values.*
> *I have good judgment.*

Add any additional qualities you think of that are not included in this list.

2. Think about all of the positive actions you have taken or are currently taking, including things you do or have done for others, your demonstrations of appreciation for others, actions you are proud of, difficult decisions you have followed through with, your accomplishments, and so on. The following examples are ideas; your list will be specific to you.

My Positive Actions

> I take good care of my children.
> I am respectful to coworkers.
> I work hard to do a good job.
> I garden.

29

I try to exercise when possible.
I watch what I eat.
I do nice things for my partner.
I take care of my things.
I play music.
I create art.
I cook well.
I help/helped_____ to_____.

Return to your PSI page, and fill in the section My Positive Actions with all of your positive actions.

3. Now ask one or two people who care about you what they consider to be your positive qualities and actions. Add these to the My Positive Qualities and My Positive Actions sections of your PSI. If you do not agree with the positive qualities or actions they note, add them to your list as that person's opinion—for example, *Sonya thinks I am helpful.*

4. Think about all of the help and support you have. Return to your PSI, and under the section titled My Positive Supports, list all of your supports. Be specific; for example, instead of writing "friends," list each friend by name. Be generous in your definition of supportive relationships, that is, even if a particular person is not always consistently supportive, consider him or her supportive for the purposes of this exercise.

Your supports do not all have to be people. They may be an activity or practice (yoga, exercise, meditation), an environment (a comfortable home, the outdoors, your workplace), cultural supports (a feeling of solidarity, community, or identity), animals, objects (cherished books that inspire you, a piece of art, photos of loved ones), or a special event or experience (a song, fond memories, a spiritual experience). Following are some examples.

My Positive Supports

friends (list each one by name)
partner/spouse
teachers
coworkers (list each by name)
supervisor
employees (list each by name)
religious community or practice

cultural or other community supports
children
relatives
music
art
gardening
nature
my home
meditation

exercise class
pets
faith
things I have learned or believe (specify) _____

_____

my skills in _____ (specify)

You have just completed your PSI. The PSI is a living list that will grow over time, as you notice and add more of your strengths and supports.

5. Now slowly read your PSI aloud to yourself—your Positive Qualities, Positive Actions, and Positive Supports. Read each item carefully enough to let it sink in. You might even want to close your eyes after you finish for a few seconds and see how you feel.

At the beginning of this exercise, I asked you to rate your positive feeling on the 0-to-10 scale. How would you rate it now? _____

When I do this exercise in my counseling practice, it is not uncommon for people to become tearful as they read the list aloud for the first time and realize all of the positives they have been overlooking. Anxiety, depression, anger, pain, loss, and stress skew our focus toward the negative. Unless we intentionally look for the positives and then deliberately focus on them, negative thoughts and feelings can take over.

But not everyone experiences an immediate difference with this exercise. If you did not notice any change in your feelings, that's OK. The way I find the PSI most helpful is to read it regularly, continue to add to it, and watch for a cumulative effect.

STRENGTHSPOTTING

If you enjoyed this exercise, here are a couple of ways to take it a bit further. The first comes from Alex Linley (Linley, Willars, & Biswas-Diener, 2010), who teaches "strengthspotting" as part of his approach to people management practices. Linley defines *strengths* as those abilities that energize you and come easily and naturally, versus abilities that come easily and naturally that are *not* energizing (which he calls *learned behaviors*).

For example, when I teach an all-day workshop, I appear to be outgoing because I engage easily with participants and genuinely enjoy the interaction. However, at the end of the day, I usually feel exhausted. In contrast, I love to write, and nothing energizes me more than a whole day of writing at home by myself. (My husband, on the other hand, hates to write; he gets exhausted just thinking about an entire day writing.) You might say that teaching is a learned behavior I've become good at with lots of practice and help from others, whereas writing is a true strength that capitalizes on my introversion. I mention this distinction here because it's one I'll come back to later, but as you're constructing your PSI, don't worry about the difference. For now, consider even learned behaviors that you are good at as strengths.

To increase your strengthspotting abilities, try some of Linley's tips:

1. Remember what you enjoyed doing as a child and still enjoy doing (because what we enjoy is often what we excel at).

2. Think about what draws your attention and interest without effort.

3. Notice what activities you excel at, that give you an energetic buzz.

4. Pay attention to activities or interests you talk about with passion, with words like "I love to . . . " and "It's great when . . . "

5. Notice what you're doing when you feel authentic, like "the real you."[1]

If you're now recognizing more of your strengths, add them to your PSI.

SIGNATURE STRENGTHS

A second way to extend your strengths focus is to check out the VIA Institute on Character (http://www.viacharacter.org/survey/Account/Register). Funded by the Mayerson Foundation, a team of social scientists studied the world's major religions, philosophies, and psychology to uncover virtues and corresponding character strengths that span human history and cultures. The team then put together a free online test that will tell you what your top five "signature strengths" are. There is nothing about weaknesses in this survey—only strengths, with a focus on pinpointing your top ones. Your survey results will also give you suggestions on ways to maximize your strengths at work and in your life. Everyone I know who has completed the test (including me) found it fun and energizing.

---

[1]Condensed from 10 tips in Linley, Willars, and Biswas-Diener (2010).

SMALL STEP

Put your PSI in a place where you will see it every day. If you live alone, post it on your refrigerator door or your bathroom mirror. If you live with others, put it in your underwear drawer, inside your appointment book, or some other place where you will see it easily and others won't.

Make a commitment to read your PSI aloud at least once a day. Think of this daily reading the way you would think about planting seeds in a flowerpot. After planting the seeds, you water the soil. The next day when you look at the flowerpot and see nothing sprouting, you don't say, "Oh, I guess it didn't work," and throw the pot away. You water the soil again, and over the next several days you continue to do so until you start to see tiny green things poking up through the soil. Your tiny green things will be those first little positive feelings and thoughts that sprout into "Maybe I *can* make a change that will stick this time."

Personal Strengths Inventory

My Positive Qualities

I am _____ .

I love _____ .

My Positive Actions

I do _____ .

I helped _____ .

My Positive Supports

(list)

Step 2:

UNDERSTANDING YOUR STRESSORS

CHAPTER 3

HOW STRESS HURTS

Stress is like an iceberg. We can see one eighth of it above, but what about what's below?

—Author unknown[1]

Stress affects you physically, mentally, and emotionally, and it even affects your relationships. Understanding the stressors in your life and how they affect you is an important step in figuring out what will help you feel better.

Now that you're actively looking for and recognizing your strengths and supports, let's take a look at what causes you stress. First of all, it is important to distinguish between *stressors* and *stress*. *Stress* refers to the *internal* feeling or condition we experience when we believe the demands of a situation are beyond our ability to cope.[2] A *stressor* is anything that *contributes to* this internal experience of stress.

The most obvious stressors are events, people, and environmental influences (including medical conditions affecting a person) that we perceive as *external* to us and mostly beyond our control. However, *thoughts* can also act as stressors because whether an event, person, or influence is stressful depends largely on how we think about

---

[1]Retrieved from http://www.stress-management-for-health.com
[2]Defined by Richard Lazarus. See http://www.universityofcalifornia.edu/senate/inmemoriam/richardlazarus.html

it. Sure, there are some external stressors (abuse, war, death, disaster) that create stress in everyone. But in most situations, it is our *thinking* that determines how much stress we actually experience.

Thoughts act as stressors in two main ways. One, thoughts can *create* stress independent of any external stressors, for example, when you make yourself sick by worrying about something that is highly unlikely to occur and out of your control anyway. Two, thoughts can *magnify* the experience of stress that comes from external stressors, for example, when someone says something hurtful to you and you go over and over it in your head for 2 days afterward. In the latter situation, the external stressor is the person's hurtful comment, and the internal stressor is your thinking (e.g., "Who does he think he is? What right does he have to say something like that? He ought to be fired"), which magnifies the hurt and anger initially caused by the hurtful comment.

In Marisol's case, her experience of stress started with a number of very real stressors in her environment: the demands of parenting two teens; impending college expenses; full-time hospital work with ill patients; and a long, traffic-filled commute to work each day. In addition, although she considered coaching her daughters' soccer team fun, it too added some stress.

A large part of these externally generated stressors were beyond Marisol's control; that is, she could not fully control the behavior of her teenagers, nor could she control the fact that college is so expensive or the amount of traffic she encountered. Although she might have considered looking for another job, for the time being she could not afford to take time off to do so. And although she could have quit the coaching position, she'd made a commitment and did not want to back out. So it is not surprising that with all of these stressors over which she had minimal control, Marisol was feeling stressed.

However, on top of these environmental stressors, Marisol was engaging in specific thoughts and ways of thinking that increased her *experience* of stress. Specifically, the more she berated herself for what she was *not* doing, as opposed to encouraging herself for what she *was* doing, the more she experienced stress emotionally (in the form of anxiety), physically (poor sleep and fatigue), and behaviorally (overeating). Her negatively skewed self-talk acted as a stressor, decreasing her optimism and energy to make positive change.

Similarly, Sheldon's environmental stressors were also big ones: the loss of his partner, a demanding job, and tighter finances with the shift from a two-person income to one. But here again, Sheldon's harsh, judgmental blaming of his former partner, supervisor, coworker, and at times himself only made him feel worse. The worse he felt, the more he behaved in ways that worked against him.

WHY WE REACT THE WAY WE DO

Wim Hof is a 52-year-old Dutch man who earned the nickname "Iceman" for his ability to withstand freezing temperatures. His accomplishments include sitting in a glass box of ice for 71 minutes on a New York City street, swimming half the length of a football field under a sheet of ice in the Arctic, and running a half marathon barefoot during subzero temperatures in Finland (Sterling & Furtula, 2011). Most people would develop hypothermia within a few minutes of exposure and die under such conditions (so don't try this at home).

Scientists found that Hof's resistance appears to be due to his ability to exercise conscious control over what we normally think of as involuntary functions, including the body's physical response to stress. Hof described his method as consisting of three elements: controlled breathing, paying attention to his body's signals, and keeping an open mind. Similar behavioral elements and effects have been found in long-term meditators. For example, in one study that compared Buddhist monks with nonmeditators of similar age, the monks had lower blood pressure, lower pulse rates, slower reaction times, and lower levels of cortisol (a hormone produced in response to stress; Sudsuang, Chentanez, & Veluvan, 1991).

But for most of us, the body's response to stress is not under our conscious control. As the neuroscientist Robert Sapolsky (2004) explained in his book, *Why Zebras Don't Get Ulcers,* humans are like the zebra when it senses an approaching lion and all of its energy goes into the huge muscular effort needed to escape. Without any conscious effort, the zebra's awareness is heightened, and its heart rate and breathing accelerate. Blood vessels dilate to increase blood flow to the muscles needed for flight while constricting elsewhere, slowing down digestive processes and sexual responsiveness. The immune system receives an immediate boost, perhaps as a counter to injuries that may occur, and the physical flight response increases the likelihood of survival.

Similarly, to ensure survival, the human brain is wired to scan for and perceive possible threats. As the saying goes, *It is safer to mistake a stick for a snake than a snake for a stick* (Love & Carlson, 2011). In reaction to an immediate stressor, the adrenal glands produce cortisol, which in turn activates antistress and anti-inflammatory pathways. A little cortisol is not a bad thing; in fact, the increased alertness and focus it brings in the short term facilitate learning and performance (which may be why some people believe they perform better under a little pressure).

But unlike the zebra, whose stress response quickly returns to normal after escaping the lion, humans have the ability to think about past threats and worry about future ones. As a result, the human stress response can get stuck on high alert, even when the threats are not physical. The accompanying high levels of cortisol can eventually suppress the immune system, leading to allergies, asthma, decreased resistance to infection, and autoimmune diseases that attack the body's own cells and tissues by mistake (e.g., chronic fatigue syndrome, fibromyalgia, thyroid disease, inflammatory bowel disease, lupus).

A prolonged stress response can also lead to high blood pressure, heart disease, insomnia, and a variety of other physical symptoms (Medline, 2013). It can exacerbate pain from an existing physiological injury or medical condition, and it can create pain as a result of prolonged muscle tension. Emotionally, persistent stress affects a person's mood, increasing irritability, anxiety, anger, fear, and depression. In turn, these emotions fuel self-defeating behaviors that negatively affect physical health, increase the risk of addiction, and damage relationships.

In the moment, stress is experienced in one or more of four areas. Physically, stress may be experienced as a headache, stomachache, sleep problems, muscle tension, low energy, poor appetite, intestinal problems, and a variety of other bodily symptoms. Mentally, stress takes the form of obsessive, intrusive, and negative thoughts and images. Emotionally, stress shows itself in anxiety, depression, irritability, anger, jealousy, and other unwanted emotions. And behaviorally, stress appears in the form of behaviors that are self-defeating and create conflict with others. All of these forms of stress interact with and affect one another (which is why a thought can act as a stressor and at the same time be the result of stress).

Consider This

Think of the last time you encountered a major stressor. How did you experience the stress in these four areas?

Physical _____

Mental (thoughts)_____

Emotional _____

Behavioral _____

FIGHT, FLIGHT, OR FREEZE—AND MORE

The human behavioral response to stress is also known as *fight/flight/freeze;* in the face of a threat, we protect ourselves through aggressive action, escape, or immobilization to avoid attention. But as recent research has found, there is more to the story.

A study conducted by the National Institutes of Health (Eaton et al., 2012) found that men tend to externalize their experience of stress more than women. Specifically, men are more likely than women to blame others and engage in aggressive behaviors (e.g., fight). Men are also more likely to isolate themselves and abuse substances (flight/escape behaviors). Sheldon's angry blaming of his former partner and coworkers and his increased drinking are examples of this tendency.

In contrast, women are more likely to internalize their distress, for example, going over and over negative thoughts and blaming themselves. This internalization often contributes to depression and difficulty taking action (a freeze response). Marisol's self-blame and overeating fit with this tendency.

In addition, scientists have recently recognized a fourth behavioral response that is largely healthy. The *tend-and-befriend* response involves positive social behaviors such as caretaking and enlisting the help of others. Studies have suggested a link between this behavioral response and the body's production of oxytocin, particularly in women during the stress of childbirth and breast-feeding when resources are focused on ensuring the survival of the infant. As researcher Shelley Taylor noted, it appears that oxytocin (and the closely related hormone vasopressin in men) acts as a thermostat for the adequacy of one's social support, signaling the need for increased support, then reducing the stress response when that support is established (Azar, 2011; "Shelley E. Taylor," 2010).

Consider This

Can you think of a recent situation in which you reacted with a fight, flight, freeze, or tend-and-befriend response? _____

Is one of these responses more common than the others for you? _____

A person's social standing also plays a role in the experience of stress. Harvard University researchers Jennifer Lerner and Gary Sherman (2012) investigated this effect of higher status in two studies that compared mid- and high-level government officials and military officers with a group of nonleaders in the community. In the first study, cortisol levels and self-reported anxiety were lower in the group of leaders than in the group of nonleaders. In the second study, which looked at differences *between* leaders, those with the highest rank and power had the lowest levels of cortisol and anxiety. In both studies, lower stress was explained by the greater control and greater sense of control that come with higher social status. So if you find yourself highly stressed in a position of lesser power or status, remember that part of your stress may be due to both your perception of less control (the internal part) and also the very real stress that comes with having less power.

One final point to keep in mind regarding stressors is that they are not always negative events. As strange as it may sound, positive events can also create stress. Researchers use the term *eustress* to describe stress that comes from something people enjoy, for example, getting married, having a baby, or winning the lottery. Although such events are desirable, they often involve a great deal of upheaval, unpredictability, and change that can have negative physical effects.

PINPOINTING YOUR STRESSORS

Clearly, people experience and react to stressors in their own unique ways. What constitutes a stressor for you may not be so for someone else. To understand the role of stress in *your* life, first you need to need to know what creates stress for you.

The exercise on the opposite page will help you pinpoint your *external* stressors (in subsequent chapters, we will look at how your thoughts magnify the effects of these external stressors). Note that these external stressors are only suggestions. If they do not fit for you, use the *Other* category to list yours.

GROWTH THROUGH ADVERSITY

If you have a lot of 4s and 5s in your list, take heart. Having problems is not always a bad thing. What matters is how you cope with them. This is the finding of the most comprehensive research on well-being ever conducted—an 8-decades-long study of 1,500 people since childhood who are now in their 80s or deceased (Friedman & Martin, 2011). Analyses of the lives of these individuals (who experienced the usual range of human problems and tragedies) found that hard work over a lifetime, especially work focused on something or someone beyond oneself, was predictive of a thriving, successful, and long life. *Persistence,* despite the difficulties life brings, was the greatest predictor of longevity.

Adversity helps people grow in a number of ways. Rising to a challenge brings out one's capabilities, which in turn increases a person's self-esteem. As my mother used to tell my sister and me when we didn't want to wash the dishes: It builds character. Adversity can also strengthen relationships through the giving and receiving of help, particularly when one is vulnerable. Although intense adversity often brings a period of confusion and uncertainty, the emotional upheaval can cause a person to question his or her values

Try This

1. Circle the areas of **negative** stress in your life:

    ____Conflicts with partner/spouse/child/parent
    ____Loss/death
    ____Work/unemployment
    ____Social life or lack of
    ____Health
    ____Traumatic experience/accident
    ____Finances
    ____School
    ____Family
    ____Too much to do (overscheduling)
    ____Community/society (e.g., racism, homophobia, and other forms
    of prejudice and discrimination)
    ____Major move
    ____Legal problems
    ____Other_____
    ____Other_____
    ____Other_____

2. Circle the areas of **positive** stress in your life

    ____New partner/spouse
    ____Birth of a child
    ____Graduation
    ____A new (desired) job
    ____Children leaving/not leaving home
    ____Retirement
    ____Winning the lottery/inheritance
    ____Fun travel
    ____Other_____
    ____Other_____
    ____Other_____

3. Using a scale from 1 (*mild*) to 5 (*major*), rate the level of stress you
experience for each stressor on the line preceding it.

and purpose in life. Embedded in this questioning is an opportunity to rethink one's goals and focus on those that increase well-being (Haidt, 2006).

Even intense adversity in the form of trauma can build a person's internal resources. For example, about one third of people exposed to a traumatic event (e.g., earthquake, hurricane, sexual assault) or chronic trauma over time (e.g., childhood abuse, war) develop posttraumatic stress disorder (PTSD). But this means that two thirds of people who experience the same trauma never develop PTSD. And of those who do develop the disorder but move through the pain to heal, the experience of being a stronger and better person than before is not uncommon. Psychologists call this phenomenon *posttraumatic growth.*

So, in sum, what really matters is not so much the number or even the intensity of stressors in your life as your reaction to these stressors. Fortunately, we have the power through our thoughts and behavior to shape and change our reactions in ways that keep us on the path of well-being.

SMALL STEP

Pick one of the stressors you rated as a 4 or 5. Throughout your day or week, watch for your reaction to this stressor, including the effects on your body, mind, behavior, and relationships. Pay attention to the part of your reaction that feels involuntary or automatic, such as an emotion or behavioral response, and the part that involves you deliberately saying or doing something (or not). If you want to maximize the usefulness of this step, keep a journal or notebook to record what you learn.

CHAPTER 4

THE MIND–BODY CONNECTION

Energy flows where attention goes.
—Michael Beckwith, founder of the
Agape International Spiritual Center

Your body is a significant source of information about well-
being, but stress can create a disconnection between your body
and mind. Mindfulness can help you reconnect and hear your
body's messages regarding your needs.

Ever since I can remember, I have always been more interested in
academic, social, and spiritual pursuits than in physical exercise. I
didn't learn how important it is to pay attention to my body until
I went through a painful divorce at the age of 37. At the time, my
main coping strategy was to immerse myself in work, which consisted of writing my first book. Working in the most uncomfortable positions on an ergonomic nightmare of a laptop, I ignored the
twinges, aches, and pains until they turned into real physical damage and the diagnosis of carpal tunnel syndrome and epicondylitis.
Looking back, I now see that my body was screaming at me, "STOP
WORKING!" but I refused to listen.

It took me several years to get back the use of my hands and
arms without pain (although I still use a voice-activated computer).
Along the way, I learned what a rich source of information the body
is regarding stress. I've even come to agree with those psychologists

49

who consider the body to be the "unconscious"—the part of us that senses and knows things that the conscious mind is unaware of. Whether you agree with this idea or not, paying attention to the physical part of yourself can have enormous benefits, even beyond physical fitness and strength.

THE ILLUSION OF MULTITASKING

The world we live in today doesn't make paying attention easy. With e-mail, texts, Twitter, Facebook, television, radio, work, household responsibilities, and relationships all competing for our attention, multitasking may seem like the logical and only possible solution. But unfortunately, for many daily tasks, multitasking doesn't work. Yes, there are some forms of information the brain can pay attention to simultaneously; for example, when you meet a new person, you are able to pay attention to multiple facial features, voice, and body language, all of which affect your response. Similarly, there are brain-directed activities people engage in simultaneously, for example, singing and playing a musical instrument. And the brain can engage in all sorts of involuntary functions (e.g., breathing) in conjunction with voluntary action.

However, the brain has more difficulty with other kinds of simultaneous tasks. For example, if you talk on your cell phone and drive, studies show that you miss more than 50% of the visual cues spotted by attentive drivers. While talking on the phone, you are more likely to have an accident than anyone else except drunk drivers, because you hit the brakes a half second slower (and in a half second, a car going 70 mph travels 51 feet; Medina, 2008).

When we engage in multiple activities such as talking on a cell phone and driving, it may *feel* as though we are multitasking. But in reality, the brain is switching attention so quickly that we only *appear* to be attending to more than one thing at once. The switching process is a little faster for younger people and familiar tasks, but it still takes time. In addition, the interruptions involved in switching decrease the quality of task performance. Studies have shown that interruptions result in 50% more errors and 50% more time to complete a task (Medina, 2008). So the teenager who has music playing, and Facebook and five other windows open on his computer while he writes a term paper and texts his best friend, is spending more time and making more errors than he would if he did each task one at a time. (Good luck convincing your teen of this, however!)

BECOMING MORE MINDFUL

Mindfulness is the opposite of multitasking. It is a simple idea: *paying attention to the present moment without judgment.* By calling your attention to the present moment, mindfulness increases awareness of the messages your body is continually sending regarding the effects of stress on your physical, mental, and emotional health.

Studies show that mindfulness improves working memory, mental flexibility, and concentration. In addition, because mindfulness involves suspending judgment (and judgmental thinking is negative), mindfulness increases recognition of the positives in life, including those often taken for granted (e.g., a warm sweater, your cat purring, a beautiful sunset). Emotionally, mindfulness increases insight, intuition, empathy, and compassion while decreasing fear and anxiety. Because it slows you down, mindfulness keeps you from reacting out of strong emotion, which helps you behave in ways that fit your long-term goals. Finally, mindfulness positively affects physical health by improving immune system functioning and overall well-being (Davis & Hayes, 2012).

But because there are so many forces working against it, mindfulness takes effort. One of the easiest ways to experience mindfulness is by focusing on your breath, as in the exercise on the next page.

(It requires you to close your eyes, so you will need to either memorize the instructions, or ask a friend to read them aloud to you.)

Try This: Breath Focus

Sit in a comfortable chair with your feet grounded on the floor and your hands resting comfortably in your lap. (Alternatively, you can lie on your back on the floor or on a bed.) Close your eyes or simply lower your gaze to the floor. Turn your attention to your breath. Take a deep breath through your nose, and at the top of the breath, hold your breath for a count of two, then slowly exhale through your nose. Take another breath like this. Now return to your normal breathing. As you focus on your breath, notice the feeling of the air moving in through your nostrils and the air moving out through your nostrils. When you notice your attention being pulled away by noises around you or thoughts that pop into your head, gently pull your attention back to your breath without any judgment about the distractions or what you are doing. Continue to focus on your breath moving in and moving out for a few minutes. When you are ready to end the exercise, wiggle your fingers and toes, blink a little, and slowly bring your attention back into the room.

Do you feel a little more relaxed after doing this exercise? Mindfulness works to calm the human arousal system in a number of ways. When focusing on the breath or whatever is occurring in the present moment, the brain is not scanning for threats. This present focus eliminates worries (which are about the future) and regrets and grievances (which are about the past). Because every moment is predictable (i.e., another breath), one feels safe. With practice, thoughts become like passing clouds that come and go.

By enabling the mind and body to stay with an experience rather than avoid it, mindfulness teaches you that by moving *into* a painful present emotion, you can move through it and survive. Longtime meditation practitioners make the point that emotional pain is a normal part of human experience, but it is our *resistance* to the pain that creates *suffering*. This *acceptance of the pain* is key to healing, because before you can change a feeling, you have to recognize and accept that it is there:

$$\text{Pain} \times \text{Resistance} = \text{Suffering}$$

The idea that resistance to pain increases suffering applies to physical pain too. As I explained earlier, the fight/flight/freeze response leads to increased muscle tension, and if you hold tension long enough, it becomes physical pain. Fear (a form of anxiety) amplifies the experience of pain. Whether the original pain comes from an emotional reaction or a physiological injury, the pain is very real. But through mindful attention to the pain, you can decrease the muscle tension that contributes to this added experience of pain (Davis & Hayes, 2012).

As you become an observer of your experience, mindfulness changes your relationship to stressors and stress. It is as though you take a step outside of yourself, as if watching a movie, to look at your experience and reactions. This creation of distance between you and your thoughts decreases the emotional and physical suffering that makes the experience of pain feel even bigger.

LISTENING TO YOUR BODY

Mindfulness calls attention to our bodies as a rich source of information about our needs. If we pay attention to our bodies' signals, we can often eliminate or prevent a worsening of physical and emotional problems. The Buddhist monk Thich Nhat Hanh (1992) explained how: by first paying attention to the physical areas in which we hold stress, tension, and pain. He said that when we experience a hurtful interaction, we develop a sort of *internal knot*. The physical location of this knot varies, but common spots include the head, jaw, neck, shoulders, chest, stomach, and intestines. If we quickly pay attention to the knot as soon as it is tied, we can usually figure out what caused it, which helps to loosen it. However, if we ignore the knot, it will continue to grow, and the longer we ignore it, the harder it will be to untie.

The following exercise is a beginning step toward listening to your body and using its signals to understand your needs. It is not a relaxation exercise, but rather an exercise in paying attention. As with the breath focus exercise, you will need to read through the entire instruction first before trying it with your eyes closed or have a friend

---

Try This: The Mind–Body Focus

1. Begin in the same way you did with the breath focus, sitting or lying comfortably, with eyes closed or gaze lowered. Turn your attention to your breath and, for a few breaths, notice the feeling of the air moving in and out through your nostrils.

2. Now focus on the part of your body where you hold tension, stress, or pain. You may notice a difference in texture, color, vibration, or sensation in this area, or you may not notice any difference at all. With your eyes closed, turn your mental awareness toward the top of this area. Slowly walk your attention to the right side of this area, then to the bottom of the area. Continue by slowly turning your mental attention to the left side and then back to the top of the area. Now, taking a three-dimensional perspective, move your attention from the front of the area through to the back, again noticing anything there is to notice. As you do the exercise, there is no need to try to relax, because this is not a relaxation exercise; rather, it is simply an exercise in paying attention.

3. When you are ready, bring your attention back to your breath, and slowly return your awareness to your present surroundings.

---

read it to you. Whichever way you use, take at least 4 or 5 minutes to do the exercise.

People vary widely in how they describe their body's area of pain or tension (e.g., as a different color, texture, size, or no difference at all) on completing this exercise. However, nearly everyone describes feeling relaxed by the exercise (despite the instruction that it is not a relaxation exercise). This calming effect illustrates how simply *paying attention* to one's body, tension, and pain usually decreases the experience of stress.

When Marisol began paying attention to her body, she was surprised to realize how much she had "tuned out." She became more aware of the fatigue that permeated her being and of the agitated feeling in her chest and stomach right before she turned to food to calm herself. She also started noticing how much she slumped, as if carrying the world on her shoulders.

Although Sheldon had always been physically active, he rarely paid attention to the connections among his physical sensations, emotions, and thoughts. As he began to watch for his body's responses, he noticed how much tension he held in his back and shoulders. Sometimes, when under serious pressure at work, he could even feel his shoulders up by his ears. He began taking deep breaths when he noticed his shoulders were up by his ears, and this small behavior decreased his tension a little.

Carol was already aware of her tendency to hold stress in the area of her heart. When feeling overwhelmed, she experienced tightness in her chest and shortness of breath, as if someone were sitting on her chest. But as she increased attention to this area throughout the day, including times she was and wasn't feeling stressed, she began to notice triggering events for her experience of stress—in the form of her own thoughts as well as others' expectations and comments.

SMALL STEP

During the next week, practice the mind–body focus at different times during the day, including a time when you are feeling stressed or in pain and another time when you're not. Think about what your body may be trying to tell you. When you are noticing the tension or pain, you may want to ask yourself, *If my body or this particular physical spot could speak, what would it say to me?*

CHAPTER 5

DISTINGUISHING INTERNAL FROM EXTERNAL SOURCES OF STRESS

Grant me the serenity to accept the things I cannot change, courage to change the things I can, and wisdom to know the difference.
—The Serenity Prayer, Reinhold Niebuhr

Before you can eliminate stress, you need to know what is causing it. External stressors are usually the easiest to recognize, but stress is also generated internally by our thoughts. Distinguishing external from internal thought stressors is important because it steers us toward the most helpful solution.

By now, you know a little more about stress, including the difference between a stressor and the experience of stress, and the ways in which stress affects you mentally, emotionally, and physically. And you've also learned how to pay attention to your body's signals through mindfulness techniques. Hopefully by now you have pinpointed a few external stressors in your life and are paying attention to your body's reactions to these external stressors.

The next step toward well-being involves recognizing internal thought stressors.

TWO SOURCES OF STRESS

To begin, think of stress in two main categories. The first category of stress comes from sources external to you, such as a demanding boss, money problems, or relationship conflicts; these are called

external stressors. The second category of stress is generated internally by thoughts, images, beliefs, and interpretations, sometimes
(but not always) in reaction to external stressors. These are called
internal or *thought stressors.*

When external stressors can be eliminated or minimized, the
preferred solution is usually an action that does so. For example,
because soccer night was exceptionally busy and stressful for Marisol,
she and her partner agreed that this would be the night they always
ate out. Although not having to cook dinner did not completely eliminate the stress that came with soccer night, it helped to decrease it.

However, sometimes an external stressor (or the external part
of a stressor) is *not* within your control to change, or you've already
taken all the steps you can. In this case, it helps to look for thought
stressors that may be exacerbating your experience of stress.

For example, Carol initially considered her husband and daughter's "unfair" expectations to be her biggest stressor and blamed their
behavior for "causing" her angry outbursts at them. But as she began
to understand the connections among her thoughts, emotions, bodily
sensations, and behavior, her view of the problem shifted to include
her own thinking. She began to see how repeatedly blaming others
and making negative interpretations of their behavior increased her
irritability to the point of anger, which in turn led her to behave impa-
tiently. She saw how blaming others also led her to overlook any
power she had to change the situation. Recognizing her own part
in the negative interactions gave her hope that her relationships and
situation could improve, because there was something she could do
about it—she could change *her* behavior.

The tricky part about figuring out what part of your stress is
due to an external stressor and what part is due to your thinking is
that the experience of stress makes it harder to see the difference.
Negative thinking skews us toward rigid, black-and-white views
in which we might completely blame ourselves or another person.

So in any stressful situation, it helps to remember that there is usually an external part that is generated by events, people, and circumstances *and* a part of the stress that is generated internally by you.

RECOGNIZING INTERNAL THOUGHT STRESSORS

There are many externally based stressors beyond our control to fix. Sometimes, even when there is some action we *could* take, we may decide not to if the action is too difficult or the risk too great. For example, although filing a grievance against an oppressive supervisor might stop his or her harassment, you might choose not to take such action because you could be fired. It is normal to feel some stress in response to situations like this. However, you can make your stress much greater by what you tell yourself, think about, and imagine. If you review every personal flaw and mistake you've ever made, or obsess about vengeful actions you could take, you create even *more* stress for yourself, on top of the stress created by the external stressor. This internally generated stress can take one or more of the physical, emotional, mental, or behavioral forms mentioned earlier. Physically, you can give yourself a stomachache, headache, fatigue, or nervous twitch and even prevent yourself from sleeping or eating. Emotionally, you increase your frustration, irritability, and fear. As negative thought stressors fuel your physical and emotional reactions, you are more likely to behave in ways that hurt your relationships and work against your long-range goals. And as these unhelpful, unhealthy behaviors persist, your willingness and motivation to take even a small positive step decline.

To pinpoint your internal thought stressors, begin by paying attention to *specific* external stressors—the more specific the better. For example, if mornings are a stressful time for you, think about the specific events, people, and circumstances that generate stress during your mornings, such as not getting enough sleep, getting small kids ready for school, a long commute, or being late for work. Then, as you focus on the specific stressor, ask yourself what you say to yourself that increases your stress in reaction to this stressor. For example, if you're not getting enough sleep, you might be telling yourself all morning: *I am sooo exhausted. I just hate this. I know I'm going to have a horrible day. I won't be able to think straight. My presentation to the staff is going to be awful.* This creates feelings of anxiety and dread on top of the fatigue you already feel and discourages you to the point of losing the motivation you do have. In turn, your negative attitude is likely to affect your work and interactions, further increasing your experience of stress.

Returning to the situations of Marisol, Sheldon, and Carol, here are some additional examples of internal thought stressors each of them had in reaction to external stressors in their lives.

Marisol
External Stressor: My oldest daughter says she needs $100 for new soccer shoes.

Thought Stressor: *Here we go again, it's always more money. Why do I even try to get ahead? I may as well give up trying to budget because there's just no point.*

Sheldon
External Stressor: Coworker calls in sick, and I have to attend a meeting in her place.

Thought Stressor: *I am sick and tired of having to do my work and everybody else's. These people have absolutely no consideration for anybody else. All I ever do is work—my own job and that of everyone else who doesn't give a crap about this company.*

Carol

External Stressor: My daughter asks me to babysit my grandson when he is sick because she and her husband don't want to miss their work.

Thought Stressor: *And what is my work—unimportant? Yeah, just ask Mom to do it because she's always there, and nothing she does is that important. Oh yeah, and so what if she gets sick—no big deal because she doesn't really have to work anyway.*

HOW THOUGHTS INCREASE STRESS

One way to think about the relationship between internal and external stressors is to imagine a train moving along a railroad track. As the train approaches a rickety bridge over a high canyon (the external stressor), the train engine (thought stressor) kicks in: *Oh my gosh, that canyon is so deep, if I make even the smallest mistake,*

Try This

1. Think of a friend who frequently looks stressed out. Can you distinguish a part of your friend's stress that is externally generated (i.e., not created by your friend) and a part that is internally generated (created or made worse by their thinking, interpretation, or a belief they hold onto)? _____

2. Now name an external stressor in *your* life. You might want to start with one of those you listed in the previous chapter under *Pinpointing Your Stressors,* but if it is a big or general one, make it as specific as you can: _____

3. Do you recognize a thought stressor that adds to your experience of stress? _____

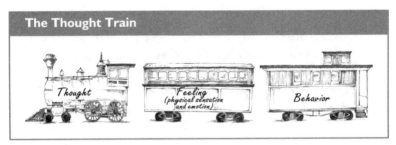

The Thought Train

Illustrations copyright 2012 by Kelsi Staton. Printed with permission.

it will all be over. I'd better not even try. This thought stressor/train engine pulls along an attached car of undesirable feelings (anxiety, fear, hopelessness, and associated physical sensations), which pulls an attached car of unhelpful, unhealthy behaviors (talking angrily to those who are trying to help you, drinking alcohol or using drugs to get through the difficult period, avoidance, or just giving up).[1]

For a day-to-day example, let's say one of your closest friends who is also your coworker moves far away. Her departure means losing your running partner, spending more time by yourself, and having some increased responsibilities at work. In reaction to this new situation, it would be normal to feel sad, lonely, hurt, irritated, or anxious. Physically, you might also experience trouble sleeping, tension in your neck, or some other symptom. Mentally, you might have difficulty concentrating and even be a little forgetful. Such reactions might affect your behavior, perhaps leading you to be less proactive about solving problems or less positive in your interactions with others.

But how you think about and interpret this loss can either minimize these emotions and behaviors or make them much worse. Returning to the train analogy, if you go over and over your neg-

---

[1]Thought train idea is from Tim Gillis, MA, LPC (personal communication, December 1, 2012).

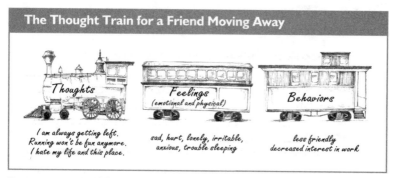

The Thought Train for a Friend Moving Away

Thoughts

I am always getting left.
Running won't be fun anymore.
I hate my life and this place.

Feelings
(emotional and physical)

sad, hurt, lonely, irritable,
anxious, trouble sleeping

Behaviors

less friendly
decreased interest in work

Illustrations copyright 2012 by Kelsi Staton. Printed with permission.

ative thoughts, telling yourself, for example, "I am going to be miserable without her, I hate my life and this place, people are always leaving and I'm the one who's left, running won't be fun anymore," these thoughts can worsen the anxiety and turn your mild irritation into anger, your sadness into depression, and your neck tension into pain. These undesirable emotions and symptoms may then increase your negative interactions with others, causing you to withdraw, increasing your loneliness and depleting the energy you have to socialize and do a good job—in short, causing a train wreck.

One last point about internally generated stress: Sometimes a thought stressor seems to pop up out of nowhere, without any obvious external stressor. For example, you might go over and over something you said or didn't say at a party, when no one else seemed bothered by your behavior, which then leads you to feel terrible and decline the next invitation. Or you might mentally rehash your anger at your former partner despite no new interactions with that person, then lash out the next time he or she calls. These thought stressors are traps that can catch you without warning, and they are the subject of our next chapter.

Try This

Think of a specific external stressor and name your reactions:

External stressor_____

Thought stressor_____

Body sensations_____

Emotions_____

Behaviors_____

Did your behavior make the external stressor worse, and if so, how?

_____

SMALL STEP

Throughout the week, when you experience a stressful situation, see if you can distinguish the part of the stress that is externally generated from the part that is internally generated by your thoughts. Write down at least one example that includes the emotions, bodily sensations, and behaviors that follow.

Step 3:

USING THOUGHTS TO FEEL BETTER

CHAPTER 6

THOUGHT TRAPS THAT CAN BLOCK YOUR PATH

"Mr. Shepherd, ye cannot stop a bad thought from coming into your head. But ye need not pull up a chair and bide it sit down."
—Mrs. Violet Brown in *The Lacuna*,
Barbara Kingsolver

Now that you understand how thoughts can increase your stress level, there are some particular thoughts to watch out for. These thought traps diminish well-being by stopping you in your tracks, and they are often so subtle that you don't even notice you're trapped.

Like a lot of people, my computer is central to my work and to my relationships. So when it does something it shouldn't, a panicky little feeling arises in me, and if I can't fix the problem immediately, a low-level anxiety nags me until I do. I know that this unwanted feeling is driven by my locomotive thoughts: *No, no, no, this can't be happening now! I don't have time for this. If only we lived in the city where it's easier to get a computer fixed. I hate this, I hate this, I hate this.*

As these thoughts fuel my anxiety, my behavior becomes more rigid and less logical. I know I can call a 1-800 number for help, and if that doesn't work I can take my computer to the shop, but instead of taking these easy steps, I spend way too much time going over and over the solutions I've already tried and fretting about "what will happen *if*."

I am fully aware that 50% of my computer-related stress is generated by my thoughts (OK, 95%), including particular ways of thinking that I call *thought traps.* Thought traps are common thoughts, beliefs, interpretations, and mental images that fuel unhelpful emotions and keep a person stuck in the same behavior that is contributing to the unhelpful thoughts and unwanted feelings. I find it helpful to divide thought traps into four main types: (a) command traps, (b) possibility traps, (c) thinking errors, and (d) script traps. Let's consider each with examples.

COMMAND TRAPS

One of the most common and powerful thought traps are the words *should/shouldn't,* along with their close cousins *have to* and *must.* If you are not doing something and you tell yourself, *I should do this, I have to do this, I must do this,* you build feelings of anxiety, hopelessness, and guilt, which in turn *decrease* your motivation to do whatever you're telling yourself you should do.

For example, if you do not want to go to a party and you tell yourself *I should want to go to this party,* the word *should* triggers additional thoughts, such as *Parties are supposed to be fun, so what is my problem? What is wrong with me?* When used in this way, these are not genuine questions, but a backhanded way of berating yourself. Such negative thoughts and feelings then further decrease any energy you have to go to the party. To paraphrase the late psychologist Albert Ellis, this is referred to as "*shoulding* on yourself."

Marisol, for instance, frequently found herself caught in a should trap, telling herself *I shouldn't feel so stressed. What's wrong with me? I should be able to cope better.* The more she repeated these thoughts to herself, the more stressed she felt, including a jittery physical feeling, nervousness, irritation, and at times even some hopelessness.

Although many people use shoulds to motivate themselves, in reality the shoulds are more likely to do the opposite. In Marisol's

---

Try This

Think of a *should* you frequently use on yourself (e.g., *I should have achieved more by now; I should know how to change a tire; I HAVE to lose weight, I shouldn't eat desserts . . .*)_____

_____

When you repeat this message to yourself a couple of times, notice any physical sensations and/or emotions. Do you feel more or less motivated to take action?_____

---

case, the more she told herself she should be able to cope better, and berated herself by asking, *What's wrong with me,* the less patient she was with her partner and kids. And the less patient she was, the worse she felt about herself, which decreased her motivation to try harder. It also left her with less energy to consider what she *could* do to decrease the external stressors over which she *did* have some control.

Another common should trap is in relation to someone else's behavior or situation, as in *He should be more considerate of me; She shouldn't talk to me that way; For everything I do for them, they should pay me more; It shouldn't be that way.* When shoulds are used toward others, they increase emotions of frustration and anger, which lead to hurtful behaviors that worsen interactions, further increasing the frustration and anger.

Sheldon was caught in the should trap regarding his former girlfriend, repeating to himself: *She should have been more understanding. She shouldn't have left me—what a #@$&!* These thoughts created a sick feeling in his stomach, tension in his neck, agitation, and anger, which led him to behave in self-defeating ways (reacting angrily toward coworkers and his boss and drinking more). As his anger elicited anger from others and the alcohol affected his reasoning abilities and self-control, he felt even angrier, which prevented him from seeing how much of his stress he was generating himself.

> ### Try This
>
> Name a *should* you think about someone with whom you have some conflict (e.g., *He should know better, She shouldn't keep doing that*)
>
> _____
>
> _____
>
> Repeat this statement to yourself a couple of times and notice any physical sensations and/or emotions. Do you feel more or less positive toward the person, more or less motivated to be helpful or generous toward them?_____

Other command-type thought traps include the words *always* and *never*. When used in relation to oneself (e.g., *I'll never be able to quit smoking/lose weight/get a better job; I always screw things up*), they diminish a person's self-esteem and increase hopelessness, anxiety, and more self-defeating behavior. When used in relation to others (e.g., *He never listens; She always wants more; He is always so stubborn; She never gives me any affection*), the words *always* and *never* increase frustration, anger, and behaviors that work against the relationship. Because *always* and *never* dismiss any possibility of the positive, when it comes to human behavior, they are not accurate, because no one behaves exactly the same way all the time. And without recognizing any possibility of the positive, they also work against healthy conflict resolution and problem solving.

POSSIBILITY TRAPS

Possibility traps focus on the future and the past. The *what-if*s increase anxiety by calling attention to an infinite number of negative possibilities: *What if the tow truck doesn't come when I need it? What if my child gets sick? What if my house burns down? What if*

I can't depend on my partner? What if I lose my job? Although the what-ifs call attention to negative events that are *possible,* the problem with them is that they simultaneously pull you away from all of the *positive* possibilities. And if you don't see any positive possibilities, your continued worrying will deplete any energy you do have to act in healthier, more helpful ways.

Similarly, the *if-only*s trap you in regret, guilt, or despair about the past: *If only I hadn't said that; If only I had worked harder in school; If only my parents had been better to me.* Here again, although these statements may be true, the problem is the exclusively negative focus that keeps you from moving forward.

Finally, the *if-then* trap can increase negative feelings by focusing on an expectation that is not or cannot be fulfilled: *If he really loved me, (then) he would remember to ask me about my day; If my workplace truly valued me, they would pay me more; If I were a better teacher, my student would not be failing the class.* The if-then trap creates frustration by perpetuating the illusion that one event automatically follows the other when this may not be the case. Using the last example, the student's failure in the class may have nothing to do with the teacher's teaching abilities. But if the teacher keeps hammering herself, she will feel worse and be less attentive to her students' needs.

Carol found herself caught in one of these thought traps, telling herself, *If my husband and daughter truly loved me, (then) they would want me to do this work that I enjoy.* As she repeated this thought, it became a belief that brought up the physical sensation of a lump in her throat and emotions of hurt, sadness, and anger. The more she repeated it, the more hurt she felt and the more she behaved negatively toward her family. With fewer positive interactions and less support from her husband and daughter, the more distant she felt from them, which then increased the belief that they did not really love her.

THINKING ERRORS

Several decades ago, the psychiatrist Aaron Beck noted what he called *cognitive errors* in his patients—inaccurate thoughts and thought patterns that contributed to mental health problems.[1] Over the years, research has shown that these errors are fundamental in creating emotional stress and fueling unhelpful behavior.

These thinking errors operate in the same way as the other thought traps. When you're using them, they increase unwanted feelings and unhelpful behavior, which increase the unhelpful thoughts that bring on more unwanted feelings and unhelpful behavior. Perfectionism is one common type of thinking error and one that Marisol struggled with in several areas of her life. For example, when she was trying to diet, at times she would overeat. She would then tell herself, *Well I've already blown it now, so I might as well eat whatever I want,* which would lead her to eat to the point of feeling sick. Then she would feel even more discouraged, making it even harder to get back on track.

Thinking errors are so common that you will probably recognize many of them in the quiz on the opposite page. You may also note that some thinking errors overlap; for example, perfectionism also includes some black-and-white thinking (e.g., *You either do it perfectly or you're a failure*).

After reading the correct answers to the quiz, go back and circle the thinking errors that most often trap you. Recognizing and changing one of these may become part of the Small Step you decide to do at the end of this chapter.

---

[1]For more on cognitive distortions, see Beck, Rush, Shaw, and Emery (1979, p. 17) and Burns (1980, p. 77).

Try This: Thinking Errors Quiz

See if you can match the following self-talk with the thinking error that best describes it.[2]

____1. Black-and-white thinking
____2. Catastrophizing
____3. Discounting the positive
____4. Mind reading
____5. Overgeneralizing
____6. Perfectionism
____7. Tunnel vision
____8. Taking things personally

A. *My spouse should know exactly how I feel about* _____ [fill in the blank].

B. *You can't trust politicians, because they are dishonest.*

C. *Either you're with me, or you're against me.*

D. That's a nice outfit. *Nah, it was really cheap, and I think it's too tight.*

E. My husband Bob, the avid fisherman: *When I don't catch a fish, I feel rejected.*

F. Student with a late paper: *If I can't get my paper done by 3 p.m., my life is over.*

G. *Show me the money, because in life, the winners are those with the most.*

H. *If you can't do it right, don't bother.*

SCRIPT TRAPS

Beginning in childhood, we all develop beliefs about the way the world works. Automatic negative thoughts and self-talk can usually be traced back to these core beliefs, most of which we hold unconsciously. These beliefs involve assumptions, rules, and expectations

---

[2]Quiz answers: 1-C, 2-F, 3-D, 4-A, 5-B, 6-H, 7-G, 8-E

that we learn through interaction with our families, our cultures, and our physical environments.

Cognitive therapists use the term *schema* to describe a set of related core beliefs. I find it helpful to think of these beliefs as a *life script,* because they guide us as we are living our lives. A life script helps us make sense of the world by influencing what we (selectively) perceive and remember and how we organize this information. Scripts affect how we think and feel about ourselves, the world, and the future, and these thoughts and feelings then affect what we do. Life scripts can be positive if they move us in the right direction, but they can also keep us trapped in self-defeating attitudes, choices, behaviors, and relationships.

When beliefs learned in childhood are reinforced by the media, peers, and cultural and religious authorities, they often influence us without our conscious awareness. For example, a child who is abused learns that she cannot trust her caregivers. As she grows up, if this belief is reinforced by negative interactions with other adults, she may develop the life script *The world is a dangerous place, and you can't depend on anyone.* If this script leads her to adopt a defensive stance in the world and withdraw from people who could love her, it will negatively affect her success in relationships, school, and work and limit her enjoyment of life.

Here are a few examples of negative life scripts:

- *Always remember, it's survival of the fittest.*
- *Don't get too happy, or something bad will happen.*
- *Expect the worst, and you will never be disappointed.*
- *I am/You are/They are not OK.*
- *Ultimately the only person you can trust is yourself.*
- *People should stick to their own kind.*
- *People will use you if you don't show them who is boss.*

Try This

1. Think of a negative message you received growing up about yourself, others, the future, or the world. If you can't think of one for yourself, think of one that someone else seems to believe. _____

_____

2. Note how this message affects your (or their):
   Attitude _____
   Emotions _____
   Choices _____
   Behavior _____
   Relationships _____

In summary, thought traps work against our happiness and well-being, largely because we do not perceive them. Once you recognize the thought traps along your path, you are in a position to avoid and eventually eliminate them. In the next two chapters, you will learn some strategies to disarm and eliminate the traps that are blocking your path now.

SMALL STEP

During the next week, watch for one of the thought traps that you tend to get caught in. If you can avoid it, great! But if not, don't worry—the first step in avoiding a thought trap is to simply become aware of it, and as you watch out for it, you will be increasing your awareness.

CHAPTER 7

COUNTERING NEGATIVE THINKING

Just keep going. No feeling is final.

—Rainer Maria Rilke

Emotions are the body–mind's warning signal that we need to make some change, but changing strong emotions when you are in the middle of them can be difficult. An easier route is often to change the way you think, which in turn can change the way you feel and behave. One of the most helpful strategies for positive thought change is *countering,* which involves questioning the truth or helpfulness of negative thoughts and replacing them with more realistic and helpful ones.

So far, we've looked at the components of well-being (positive emotions, mental and physical health, healthy relationships, and a sense of purpose) and the well-being *path* as one that involves healthy, helpful ways of thinking and behaving. Next, we considered external stressors that work against well-being and the importance of listening to your body's messages regarding the effects of these external stressors on you. Then, in the last two chapters, I explained how thoughts can become stressors themselves, particularly in the form of thought traps that create and magnify feelings of anxiety, depression, anger, guilt, and other unwanted emotions.

In this chapter, I explain how to use a tool called *countering* to change strong unwanted emotions. Countering involves questioning your negative, unhelpful thoughts and replacing them with realistically positive thoughts that build well-being.

But before trying to change a strong unwanted emotion, it is important to recognize exactly *what* you are feeling, to try to understand it, and to allow yourself to experience and constructively express it. If you try to skip this understanding/experience step by pushing down or ignoring the feeling, it can pop up when you least expect it and lead to behavior that hurts you and others. Once you recognize your feelings and allow yourself to experience the emotion, then you'll be ready to change them to more positive ones. So before getting into the details of countering, let's look at some ways to understand, experience, and constructively express emotion.

RECOGNIZING AND EXPERIENCING EMOTION

Figuring out exactly what you're feeling is important because it helps you figure out what to do. If you are feeling low in energy and a little irritated, then by paying attention to your body, you realize you are hungry and tired, and eating a sandwich and resting for a half hour may be all you need. Or if you feel hurt, maybe you need to talk to the person who hurt you or to a trusted friend who will help you feel better.

Most people have a particular emotion that dominates their response to stress. Because men tend to externalize emotional pain, their dominant emotional response is often anger, which can mask deeper, less acceptable feelings in men such as hurt, fear, disappointment, guilt, sadness, and feelings of worthlessness or powerlessness. In contrast, women tend to internalize pain, with feelings of depression masking anger, an emotion less accepted in women. Sometimes just an *awareness* of the origin of an emotion, even if you can't do anything about it in the moment, can help you feel a little better. For example, if you feel especially nervous and jittery about a presentation you're about to give, and then in paying attention to your body and emotions you remember that part of your jittery feeling is coming from the fact that you had three cups of coffee that morning, this awareness may decrease some of the worry you have about how your presentation will go.

To understand feelings and emotions, I find it helpful to remember a definition behavioral psychologists use: An *emotion* is a physical sensation that we give a particular name on the basis of the context in which it occurs. For example, if you are mentally dreading an upcoming event and experiencing the physical sensations that go with that dread (e.g., upset stomach, jitteriness, rapid heartbeat, shortness of breath), you interpret these sensations to be anxiety. However, if you experience the same sensations right before a trip you are looking forward to, you interpret the sensations as excitement. When we say we have a *feeling,* we are usually referring to a physical sensation and an emotion.

Alcoholics Anonymous has a great acronym that helps with recognizing emotions: HALTS. Before acting on overwhelming feelings, this acronym *halts* you, giving you time to ask yourself, *Am I hungry, angry/anxious, lonely, tired, sick, or sad?*

Try This

The next time you feel a strong undesirable emotion, pay attention to your body for cues regarding what the emotion is and what it is truly about. As you note your physical sensations, ask yourself, *What am I experiencing? Is this really [for example] anger, or is it something else? Am I hungry, angry, anxious, tired, sick, sad, or upset about something else?*

THE EMOTION CONTINUUM

It is helpful to think of undesirable emotions as existing on a continuum. On one end, the milder versions can be helpful because they prompt us to pay attention and make more deliberate choices (see the figure on the next page). The word *emotion* comes from the word *emote*, which means *move*, and emotion helps us move into action. For example, physical sensations such as an adrenaline rush, tightening chest, or butterflies in your stomach, are the body's way of saying, "Hey, wake up, something is going on here, and I don't like it!"

However, an extreme undesirable emotion (the opposite end of the continuum) usually has the opposite effect. Rather than motivating us to do something helpful, extreme negative emotions usually *prevent* positive action, instead contributing to a fight, flight, or freeze response.

For example, when another car is riding the rear of your car and flashing its lights at you, it is normal to feel some irritation or mild anxiety. These emotions and your physical reaction (e.g., feeling hot or agitated) call your attention to the danger of the situation and, in this case, the need for action (pulling over to let him pass). However, if you start ranting and swearing at the other driver and work yourself into a rage, your extreme emotional reaction makes it less likely you will take helpful action and more likely you will do something that makes the situation worse.

When emotions become overwhelming and persistent to the point that they impair a person's functioning, they are referred to as *disorders* (e.g., an anxiety disorder or major depression). If you think you may have an emotional disorder, a first step is a medical checkup to rule out any problems such as low iron levels or thyroid dysfunction that might contribute to the symptoms.

Although medication is often assumed to be the treatment of choice for emotional disorders, research has shown that cognitive

Emotion Continuum		
Mild	**Moderate**	**Extreme**
├──────────────┤──────────────┤		
irritation	anger	rage
├──────────────┤──────────────┤		
embarrassment	guilt	humiliation, shame
├──────────────┤──────────────┤		
disappointment	sadness, normal grief	depression, hopelessness
├──────────────┤──────────────┤		
anticipation, mild worry	fear, anxiety	terror
├──────────────┤──────────────┤		
mild envy	jealousy	extreme jealousy

and behavioral interventions are often equally effective without side effects. Regarding the question of whether to use a psychiatric medication, I find this saying helpful: *Medication is the life ring they throw you when you fall in the river. It keeps your head above water, so you don't drown; but you still have to learn how to swim.* Learning how to swim involves changing what you do and how you think (using the tools described herein). Because emotional disorders skew a person's thinking so much toward the negative, if you think you may need medication, I recommend seeing a psychologist or counselor who can help you figure out the best course of action, and in conjunction with a medical provider, figure out whether medication might help.

EXPRESSING EMOTIONS CONSTRUCTIVELY

Before we move into changing negative thoughts, there is still one more important point to be made regarding emotions. Once you recognize what you're feeling, it is equally important that you allow yourself to experience it. If you try to get out of experiencing an emotion via avoidance, stuffing, or using some substance to suppress it, it will usually pop up later without an invitation.

For example, I once worked with a woman who was an expert at positive self-talk. She was single, worked full-time, and supported a child with a disability. She grew up in foster homes and had learned to put on a happy face no matter what. Her attempt to be positive was helpful in some ways; however, she would not allow herself to feel the mixture of pain, grief, and anger over the loss of her husband and worry over the obstacles that her child faced. As quickly as these feelings started to surface, she would push them down with positive self-talk but then suffered from anxiety, chain smoked, and snapped at the people she supervised.

When you need to express emotion, *constructive* expression is key. Take anger, for example. There are a couple of different approaches to constructively expressing anger. For people who tend to push anger down, hold it in, and try to ignore it, the best approach involves mindful attention to and acceptance of the internal experience of emotion (e.g., with the mind–body exercise described in Chapter 4), followed by external expressions of anger. For example, people who grow up in abusive, alcoholic, or drug-addicted homes have often learned that it is not OK to talk about feelings or, for that matter, to even *have* feelings. So what they need first is to recognize and accept these emotions, experience them, and express their pain.

Many of the strategies for constructively expressing emotions are those that children figure out on their own, for example, stomping around outside, throwing rocks into a pond, drawing and painting angry pictures, listening to music that matches your mood, yelling and crying into a pillow, or talking to a trusted person such as a friend or therapist who will validate your feelings. Anything physical that does not hurt anyone or anything is usually a good release—for example, going to the beach and shouting into the wind, working out, or running. Research has shown that writing is also a powerful release and intervention in itself, in part because it helps a person organize and make meaning out of his or her experience.

The second approach to expressing anger works better for people who focus on and externally express their anger too much. If this is your style, then you may have noticed that the more you express your anger, the bigger it gets, to the point that you might even physically hurt yourself or someone else. The best solutions for this kind of anger involve mindfulness exercises that help you become more accepting of the internal experience of emotion, followed by the use of thought-change tools and actions to let go of and calm the anger.

Consider This

Which approach to anger do you tend toward? _____

COUNTERING NEGATIVE THINKING TO FEEL BETTER

First of all, not all unwanted emotions can or ought to be changed. Anger, irritation, fear, disappointment, and sadness may be normal reactions to a situation. For example, if someone you love dies and you feel grief, the grief signifies the importance of that person to you; if you didn't feel it, you wouldn't be human, so it isn't healthy to try to get rid of it.

The problem comes in when emotions become overwhelming, and in desperation you either give up trying and become avoidant or try so hard to gain control that you make quick, poor decisions and engage in behavior that feels good in the moment but works against you in the long run. These overwhelming emotions that you have created by your thinking are the ones that thought-change tools are intended to change.

The thought train (see Chapter 5) is a handy way to explain how thoughts lead to particular feelings and behaviors; however, there is some debate regarding whether the thought always creates the feeling. It may be that sometimes the physical sensation occurs first, and then our mental interpretation of it determines the emotion (e.g., when someone startles you, you physically flinch, then feel fear). Whichever is the case, most psychologists agree that thoughts, feelings, and behaviors are so interconnected that if you change one, you'll probably get a change in the others. But directly changing a strong emotion is very difficult. (The next time you're really mad, try to "Stop feeling angry, and just BE happy!") An easier route is usually changing your thinking, behavior, or environment, which in turn then changes the emotion.

Countering is one of the most effective tools for eliminating the negative thinking that undermines well-being. As I mentioned earlier, it involves questioning negative, unhelpful, and unrealistic thoughts, then replacing them with more positive, realistic, and helpful ones. There are two kinds of countering. The first kind consists of questioning the *truth* of your thoughts, with the following kinds of questions.

Truth Counters:

- Is this thought, belief, or statement *true?*
- Who says it is true? Is it a message or norm from my family, culture, authorities, or peers? If yes, is it one I want to hold onto?
- What is the evidence that it is true? What is the evidence that it is not?

Truth counters can be very effective in eliminating thought traps and negative scripts, particularly when you are telling yourself untruths. For example:

Thought Stressor: *When it comes to getting this really great job, I know I don't have a chance.*

Truth Counter: *Who says I don't have a chance? Is anyone telling me this besides myself? Where's the evidence that I have no chance? And if I don't get this one, who says I won't get a different one that's even better?*

But truth counters don't work for all kinds of negative thinking, particularly when the thought *is* true. For example, if your house is a mess and you keep saying to yourself, *This house is a mess,* it won't help to insist to yourself that your house is really looking good. In these situations, it is more helpful to counter the helpfulness of the thought—for example, asking yourself, *Does it really help or motivate me to keep repeating this to myself?* Because helpfulness counters work for both true and untrue thoughts, I use them a lot more, myself.

Helpfulness Counters:

- Even if it is true, is it *helpful* to keep repeating this thought to myself, holding onto this belief, or focusing on this image?
- Is there a more helpful, balanced, or positive way to say it?

Like truth counters, helpfulness counters open the way for more positive, realistic, and helpful *replacement* thoughts—often in the form of responses to your questions. Regarding the messy house, your positive replacement would probably sound something like: *I know the house needs cleaning but I can't do it right now, so is it helpful to keep hammering myself with what a mess it is?* To think of the most convincing positive replacements, imagine what you would tell your best friend or child if they were in a similar situation or what they would tell you. For example:

Positive Replacement: *It would be nice if you could clean your house, but you have too much on your plate right now. In the larger picture, it's really not the most important thing. Just do some little thing, like clean the bathtub next time you're taking a shower, and then the next day, do some other little thing, and then forget about it the rest of the time. Nobody ever died of a messy house. What's the worst that could happen if you don't clean your house for another month?*

Try This

When you have difficulty thinking of helpful self-talk, ask yourself, *What would I say to my best friend or child if they were in this situation, or what would they tell me?*_____

Putting this all together, remember when Marisol's daughter told Marisol she needed $100 for new soccer shoes? In response to this kind of request (which was an external stressor for Marisol), Marisol's typical pattern was that she would experience a feeling of fatigue wash over her, followed by an empty sensation in her stomach and the emotion of anxiety. She would then think, *Why do I even try to get ahead? I may as well give up trying to budget because there's just no point.* The more she focused on these thoughts, the more hopeless she felt, which triggered even more negative thoughts, including her thought trap, *I shouldn't be so stressed. What is wrong with me?* which implied that she was not an OK person. These thoughts and feelings created a strong urge to soothe herself, which led her to eat a candy bar, then another candy bar.

Although eating the candy temporarily filled the empty feeling in her stomach and calmed her anxiety a little, as soon as she was done, she felt guilty. She then mentally beat herself up (more negative thoughts) about eating the candy and turned her initial mild guilt into a feeling of shame. (Psychologist Steven Hayes noted that the difference between guilt and shame is that guilt is the recognition and thought *I've done something bad,* and shame adds the thought *and because I did something bad,* I'm *bad.* [Hayes, 2008]) The shame Marisol then felt about her overeating, her weight, and herself further eroded her hope and energy to make any positive change.

But as Marisol began to take a more understanding approach to her emotional well-being, she became more aware of this pattern. She recognized a number of external stressors that were contributing to her general level of stress, and she could see how, in response to her daughter's simple request, she had made her experience of stress even greater. She began to notice when she was being pulled into her self-defeating pattern and to use the countering technique to stop its powerful pull.

In response to this particular stressor of her daughter's request, when she first noticed the fatigue and empty stomach sensations, she took a deep breath and began questioning the truth of what she was saying to herself.

> **Truth Counters:** *OK, what's going on here? Is this really all about money? Is budgeting really pointless? And who says I shouldn't feel stressed?*

As she learned more about countering, Marisol also began countering the helpfulness of her thoughts.

> **Helpfulness Counters:** *Yes, I'm feeling stressed, but is it helpful to keep asking myself what's wrong with me, when it's really just a way to hammer myself?*

These kinds of questions opened Marisol to helpful replacement thoughts, which were also more realistic and gave her more energy and hope that she could change.

> **Positive Replacements:** *I'm feeling stressed because I have a lot of responsibility. I'm trying to be a good mom and responsible about money. I'm doing my best, but maybe I need something more? Yes, I need to find some better ways to comfort myself than eating, and I need to decrease the stressors in my life. I've taken a good first step with my monthly walk in the woods. I'm not ready yet to start a diet, but I'm going to stop beating myself up about my weight and focus instead on building my energy and willpower by thinking more positively and continuing to take small steps.*

Try This

1. Name an external stressor and the physical sensations and emotions it brings up in you.
   External stressor: _____
   Physical sensations: _____
   Emotions: _____
2. Write a negative thought or belief that increases these unwanted physical sensations and emotions: _____
   _____
3. Now write a realistic truth or helpfulness counter that helps you feel a little better. If you have difficulty coming up with one, think of what you would say to your best friend or child or what they would tell you:
   _____
   _____
4. As you say this more positive, helpful thought to yourself, how do you feel?
   _____

SMALL STEP

Throughout the week, whenever you notice the external stressor, physical sensations, and/or related emotions, try practicing your truth or helpfulness counter and watch for a change in how you feel.

CHAPTER 8

COMPASSION VOICE

If we make friends with ourselves, then there is no obstacle to opening our hearts and minds to others.

—Author Unknown[1]

The harsh, critical voice inside our head prevents us from moving ahead; diminishes the enjoyment of our success; and keeps us stuck in an unhappy, unhealthy place. *Compassion voice* is a tool that counters this judgmental voice and replaces it with thoughts, feelings, and behaviors that feel good and are good for us.

There is a story about a wise Indian elder who was teaching his grandson about life. The elder told his grandson, "In my head, as in every person's, there are two dogs, and these dogs are at war with one another. One dog is a mean dog that is full of anger, hatred, fear, self-pity, greed, and arrogance. The other dog is a kind, loving dog—generous, peaceful, humble, faithful, truthful, and compassionate. Every day these two dogs are at war with each other." The grandson thought for a minute, then said, "Tell me, Grandfather, which dog will win?" to which the grandfather replied, "The one I feed."

Most of us are aware of the critical, judgmental voice in our head that drags us down and makes us feel terrible—a voice that

---

[1]Retrieved from http://www.thinkexist.com

dominates when we're angry, anxious, jealous, or depressed. One of the most powerful tools for countering this unhelpful voice is what I call *compassion voice*—the voice that opens your heart and mind to the positive possibilities in yourself and others.

Compassion voice is not passive or milk toast. It does not grant you permission to indulge in every urge and impulse. Rather, it is a proactive voice that counters your harsh, judgmental voice with realistic self-talk that recognizes problems but also acknowledges your strengths, supports, and positive possibilities. It is the voice you use when talking to a young child or dear friend who feels terrible about something—even if they created the problem—to help them feel better and move forward. It is the voice that guides you toward healthy choices that may take a little more effort in the here and now but be the best for you in the long run. Strengthening your compassion voice—toward yourself and toward others—can help you feel better, be more at peace, and improve your relationships.

COMPASSION VERSUS JUDGMENTAL

Have you ever noticed how many times in a day you make judgments? *Is this a healthy meal or an artery clogger? Does this outfit work for me, or should I give it up? Should I follow my heart's desire or wait a little while?* Judgments are a necessary part of living, and when they guide us toward healthy choices and behaviors, they help us and those around us. But when judgments become *judgmental,* they make our lives difficult.

The difference between *making a judgment* and *being judgmental* is that judgments are aimed at solving a problem or making a decision, whereas judgmental thoughts, words, and actions contain a superior, shaming tone: *If they weren't such idiots, they'd know how to do it; I should be better/smarter/faster than this; This is ridiculous—no one should have to put up with this crap.* (Notice the thought traps in these statements.) The judgmental voice skews a person so far toward the negative that it prevents a realistic understanding of oneself, others, and situations (as there are always positive possibilities in any person or situation). This overly negative skew works against constructive problem solving and the enjoyment of success and disconnects us from others.

In contrast, when you think compassionate thoughts, these thoughts create a compassionate feeling that inspires compassionate behavior (a positive form of the thought train). For example, think about holding a week-old puppy, its softness, warmth, and vulnerability—it's a good feeling, right? This feeling inclines you to be gentle with the puppy, even when he eats your shoe.

When you are in compassion mode, you can still make constructive judgments regarding others—for example, when someone you love does something unhealthy or hurtful and you know (i.e., judge) that it is not good, but you still care about the person. (In contrast, when you are feeling judgmental, compassion disappears.) The caring acceptance that comes with compassion allows you to see situations, yourself, and others for how and what they truly are—the positives as well as the negatives.

Try This

For 1 hour, pay attention to the number of judgments you make regarding whether something is good or bad, safe or unsafe, interesting or boring, expensive or cheap, beautiful or ugly, wise or unwise, fast or slow, important or unimportant, worthwhile or not. Notice whether your intention/tone is understanding or judgmental.

BUILDING YOUR COMPASSION VOICE

Although we usually think of compassion as a way of feeling toward others, if you want to be more compassionate toward others, it is equally important to think compassionately about yourself. But self-compassion can be challenging, as we are bombarded on a daily basis with judgmental messages from work environments, the media, and so-called authorities that we are not stylish enough, thin enough, quick enough, flexible enough, funny enough, tough enough, and the list goes on. Sometimes these messages selectively merge with negative beliefs and thoughts we have internalized from childhood, adding to or reinforcing negative life scripts.

The critical, judgmental self-talk that comes out of negative life scripts can erode your sense of self-worth, and the worse you feel about yourself, the less energy you have for anyone else. So let's look at some ways to build compassion toward yourself, which in turn will help you become more compassionate toward others.

INCREASING SELF-COMPASSION

You might believe that self-compassion equals self-indulgence, but in fact, studies have found the exact opposite. People who practice self-compassion are more able to minimize their stress because they do not get caught in a self-berating thought trap that fuels guilt, avoidance of the problem, and self-defeating behavior. They are more able to face the stressor head on, to realistically recognize how they may be increasing their stress, and then change their thinking and behavior in helpful ways.

For example, in a study conducted by researcher Mark Leary (Adams & Leary, 2007), female participants were invited to eat doughnuts for a taste-test experiment. One group of the women were prompted beforehand with self-compassion statements such as "Everyone eats unhealthy sometimes, and everyone in this study eats this stuff, so I don't think there is any reason to feel really bad about it" (Adams & Leary, 2007, p. 1129). Later, these same women were asked to taste test a number of candies. Of the women who identified themselves as frequent dieters or guilty eaters, those who had been primed by the self-compassion statements ate less candy than those who were not given the self-compassion prompt.

These results suggest that if people are kinder to themselves about their overeating (i.e., do not beat themselves up about it), they do not experience as much guilt and are more likely to eat with intention rather than overeat even more. So judgmental self-talk such as *My thighs look like saddlebags, and if I keep eating like this I'll be mistaken for a horse* will not help you stick with a diet as effectively as compassionate self-talk that recognizes the challenges and addresses them in an encouraging way.

Along the same lines, in a series of studies investigating the relationship of self-compassion to negative events (e.g., an unflattering evaluation by others or poor performance on a task), participants who were *high* in self-compassion were actually *more* likely to consider how their behavior or personality may have contributed to the unflattering evaluation or their poor performance (Leary, Tate, Adams, Allen, & Hancock, 2007). Self-compassionate individuals did not blame themselves in an obsessive way, but rather they were less defensive, which then helped them see what they could improve in themselves for the future. This lesser defensiveness reflects self-compassionate individuals' greater acceptance of themselves, including their own weaknesses and failures.

To increase compassion voice toward yourself, I have found three helpful strategies, which are described as components of self-compassion by researcher Kristin Neff (2011). The first is to take a kind and understanding approach to yourself regarding your emotions and behaviors, even the ones you don't like. Trying to understand yourself in a caring way eliminates the defensiveness that can prevent you from seeing your part in your stress and opens you to possibilities for positive change. This understanding is important, because in order to change a behavior, first you have to understand what purpose or function it serves or used to serve but now no longer does.

For example, I once worked with a young woman who cut her arms when she was upset, then afterward would quickly dismiss her behavior with the statement (which she repeated to herself and me), "Oh, I know I am so stupid to do that." This statement appeared to be an explanation for her behavior (i.e., "I did it because I am stupid"), but in reality it was just a way to avoid a difficult topic. It was not until she began trying *nonjudgmentally* to understand why she hurt herself—what purpose and function it was serving for her—that she could look for other ways to meet this need and permanently change the behavior.

When Sheldon began paying attention to his self-talk, he could see how hard he was on himself and that the more negatively he judged himself, the less patience he had for others. As he nonjudgmentally began to question why he was so hard on himself, he realized that some of his thoughts and behaviors were driven by beliefs that he had developed as a child. Bullied for being overweight and wearing thick glasses, he coped by pouring himself into his schoolwork and then later his career. His hard work was rewarded with good grades and praise from teachers and employers. He eventually lost the weight and obtained contact lenses, but his belief that "people love you for what you do" persisted, and he continued, as his former girlfriend said, "to work like a dog."

With the help of his mom and new friend Joe (whom he met at basketball, which he had started playing again once a week as his first small step), Sheldon began to counter his belief and related thoughts with the understanding and encouraging statements his mom and Joe said to him: "Your girlfriend left you because she wanted to spend more time with you—she cared about *you*, not your production capacity. You need to give yourself some slack, have more fun. If you want to be happy, you can't just work, work, work."

Putting their words into his own, Sheldon's compassion voice told him, *Melia left because she wanted to spend more time with me—not with what I did. It's too late with her, but I've got my folks, Joe thinks I'm a good guy, and the basketball guys like me to hang out with them. I really don't have to get this report done tonight. I'll have more energy to do it tomorrow if I kick back tonight.* These new thoughts did not immediately eliminate Sheldon's critical self-judgments, but as he repeated the compassionate thoughts to himself over time, he was more able to let go of self-imposed deadlines and increase his leisure time a little more.

The second way to increase self-compassion is to recognize your common humanity, which involves thinking about your personal experience in a way that connects you to others. For example, if you make a mistake, compassion voice acknowledges your good intentions and says that you are not the only one who makes mistakes or has this problem. Thinking of yourself and your situation in this way decreases the feeling of isolation (and isolation is linked to

---

Try This

1. Think of a quality, characteristic, or behavior of yours that you beat yourself up about: _____

2. Write a nonjudgmental, understanding, but realistic compassion voice alternative. If you have difficulty thinking of one, imagine what someone who loves you would say:_____
   _____

3. Do you notice a different feeling when you use your compassion voice?

---

anxiety and depression). It can also help your relationships directly if you use your experience to help someone else. As my mom used to tell me when I was hurt by a classmate's teasing or being picked last for sports teams, "Remember how it hurt, and down the road, you can use your experience to help someone who is hurt by this kind of experience too."

In Sheldon's case, it was encouraging for him to know that Joe had been through a divorce, then met someone new and was now pretty happy with his life. Sheldon added the following to his compassion voice: *OK, I'm not the only one who's been through a breakup. Joe went through a divorce, he was married way longer than I was with Melia, and he survived. And at least three of the seven people at work have been divorced too.*

The third way to increase self-compassion voice is through increased mindfulness, that is, a willingness to see things as they really are (including yourself) rather than what you wish them to be. The willingness to see yourself as you truly are allows for a realistic assessment of your contribution to your stress, which is the part you can change. It is what distinguishes a "woe is me" self-pity that leads to inaction or destructive behavior from healthy self-compassion and behavior that points you toward well-being. For Sheldon, increased mindfulness meant becoming more aware of how much he was blaming others and thinking more about what he did in the relationship that contributed to the break-up.

> **Consider This**
>
> Is there a stressor in your life for which it could help to remind yourself that you are not the only one who has made this mistake or has this problem?

USING YOUR PERSONAL STRENGTHS INVENTORY

One additional way to increase self-compassion is to use your Personal Strengths Inventory (PSI) in a way that works for you. In Sheldon's case, writing his strengths and supports in the form of the PSI called his attention to qualities (not just his work accomplishments) that he could use as part of his compassion voice (e.g., *The guys at basketball think I'm funny; A couple people at work keep asking me to go out with them, so they must like me; I know I'm smart and a hard worker*). When Sheldon noticed the tension in his neck and shoulders—his body's signal that he was feeling pressured, discouraged, or lonely—he'd remind himself of these strengths and supports to help himself feel more hopeful.

Carol used her PSI in a different way. She was an oldest child who, growing up, had to take care of her siblings because her mother was alcoholic and her father left them without support. As a result, she had internalized the message *It's all up to you, there's no else to take care of your brothers/sisters/mom; if you don't do it, everything will fall apart.* This belief led her to give such disproportionate attention to the needs of others that she neglected her own.

Initially, when Carol began making her PSI, it was hard for her to recognize her own strengths and supports by herself. However, when she asked her husband, daughter, siblings, and friends what they considered her strengths, they gave her enough to create a long list. To build her self-confidence and a new belief that she too deserved to be cared for, she decided to read her PSI aloud to herself daily and add one new strength or support per week. If she did not entirely believe one of the strengths that someone told her about herself, she would say, for example, *Jenny thinks I'm smart.*

To counter her belief that everything would fall apart if she didn't do "whatever," she included individuals (friends, family members, coworkers), groups, and environments (e.g., church, workplace) that could and would help her if she asked. Actively looking for strengths and supports to add to her list took up the time and energy she had been using to berate herself about what she was not doing. As a result, her self-confidence grew and she had more energy to interact positively with her family even when they disagreed.

COMPASSION TOWARD OTHERS

As the Dalai Lama (Dalai Lama & Cutler, 2009) has noted, disconnection from others is one of the greatest sources of unhappiness. Using your compassion voice about others can help you be happier and improve your relationships by countering the judgmental, negative thoughts that fuel negative feelings that push people away. It can help you stay open to difficult people, to see their humanness, even if you do not like what they do. And the feeling of compassion is a lot more enjoyable than irritation, anger, and judgmental thoughts.

Try This

1. Think of someone who angers or irritates you. Name two things this person does or two characteristics of theirs that you dislike:

   _____

   Name the feeling these thoughts create in you, including any desire to move away from or toward this person:

   _____

2. Now think of someone you love and a time they did something especially wonderful for you:

   _____

   Name the feeling these thoughts create in you, including a desire to move toward or away from this person:

   _____

The word *compassion* comes from the Latin *cum patior*, meaning to suffer with. This empathy for another person is the opposite of *apathy*, meaning not suffering or caring (Barasch, 2009). One of the quickest ways to feel more compassionately toward another is a strategy I call *imagine suffering*. With this approach, you try to learn as much as possible about the person to see them as a whole human being who experiences pain and suffering too. If you don't know enough about the person to know how they suffer, try guessing at the possible pain in the person's life. Keep in mind that underlying most expressions of anger is hurt.

Marisol used this strategy to get along better with one of the administrators at the hospital where she worked. She knew that the administrator, Anya, was single and had recently moved to the area for her job. What bothered Marisol was that Anya was quick to point out mistakes but did not comment on what Marisol did well. This persistent negative feedback added to Marisol's judgmental self-talk, anxiety, and feelings of hopelessness.

To decrease her irritation, Marisol used her compassion voice to tell herself, "Anya's new, so she probably doesn't have any friends here, she's probably really lonely, and when she points out mistakes, she's probably just trying to do what she thinks is her job because she's never had anybody teach her that good managers give more positive feedback than negative." Repeating this message to herself helped Marisol feel sympathetic toward Anya, which led Marisol to ask Anya questions about herself. This simple act of reaching out to Anya created a warm feeling between them, and Anya became a little more positive in her interactions.

The second tool I use a lot is what I call the *most generous interpretation* technique. Here's how it works. When we do something hurtful or wrong, we tend to explain our actions in the most generous possible way: "I know I shouldn't have used that nasty tone with him, but I was just tired/needed a break/was feeling overwhelmed/

was frustrated to the max." In contrast, when someone does something hurtful or wrong to *us,* we often think of their action with the least generous explanation: "He used that nasty tone because basically he's a jerk." The most generous interpretation involves applying the compassion voice we use to explain our own behavior to the behavior of others.

Sheldon inadvertently learned how to do this following an experience with a coworker who was driving a company truck with Sheldon in the passenger seat. Sheldon hadn't known the coworker previously, and during the course of their ride, the coworker made several driving mistakes apparently without awareness. Sheldon's irritation increased to anger as he repeated to himself what an idiot the driver was, how incompetent he was, and so forth. Sheldon didn't say anything to the coworker, but later when talking to the coworker's supervisor, he angrily told the supervisor about the mistakes. The supervisor responded, "You know, Sheldon, Keo is basically a good worker, but he's got a lot on his plate right now, and he's new to this kind of work. I'm guessing we didn't give him enough training time. I'll follow up and be sure he gets the help to learn what he needs to know." The supervisor's compassionate response suddenly deflated Sheldon's puffed up feeling of anger. As Sheldon considered the supervisor's response, he realized how much better it felt to think of the driver in this kinder way and not be angry.

A third way to increase compassion toward others is a variation of the PSI, namely, actively looking for the strengths in others (or *strengthspotting,* to use Alex Linley's term as discussed in Chapter 2). Looking for the strengths in others creates positive feelings in you and them, whether you use their strengths as part of your compassion voice toward them (e.g., "Yes, she screwed up but she thought she was doing the right thing, and she really is a hard worker") or you point out a person's strengths aloud to them in the form of compliments.

Looking for others' strengths works best when you look for specific strengths, not just "She's really nice" or "He's a good guy." My husband, Bob, told me a story that's a reminder of what not to do in this regard. He was working as a supervisor of a school principal who was pretty negative. Not surprisingly, the teachers were not happy with the principal, and Bob advised him to start giving the teachers more positive feedback. So the principal wrote on a sheet of paper, "You're doing a good job," made 20 copies of the paper, and put it in all of the teachers' boxes. Needless to say, it did not help the principal's case with the teachers.

SMALL STEP

During the next week, use your compassion voice with yourself or toward someone you consider difficult. When you are thinking more compassionately, watch for changes in your feelings and behavior.

CHAPTER 9

WELL-BEING BOOSTERS

The secret to happiness is not having what you want; it is wanting what you have.

—Buddhist saying

> Countering and compassion voice are the basic tool set for changing unhelpful thinking, and their effectiveness can be increased with these six *well-being boosters* that increase positive emotion, helpful behavior, and healthy interactions with others.

I think of countering and compassion voice as the basic tools for changing unhelpful thinking; in this chapter, I add the following as extras to make the tools work even better. Or as my handyman husband, Bob, said when I explained this idea to him, "Like when I need to tighten a nut, I can choose a vice grip, an open-end wrench, a closed-end wrench, locking jaw pliers, or a needle nose." There were several more options, but he lost me after the open-end wrench, and I'm not sure I like the nut analogy, but you get the idea: These well-being boosters will expand your toolkit.

As you use these six tools, remember that you are the expert on you. If a tool doesn't work for your particular situation, adapt it to fit your needs or try a different tool, because not every tool fits every problem, or every person. Keep in mind the *path of least resistance* principle, and start with the one that's easiest for you to increase the likelihood that the tool will work and that you will stick with it.

I. ATTITUDE OF GRATITUDE

Expressing gratitude is one of the most powerful happiness producers over time. In a study conducted by gratitude researcher Robert Emmons and his colleague M. E. McCullough (2003), participants who listed five things they were grateful for each week for 6 weeks felt more optimistic and satisfied with their lives than control groups of people who thought about five daily hassles or major events. Relative to the control groups, the gratitude group also reported fewer physical symptoms (e.g., headache, acne, coughing, nausea) and they spent more time exercising. Sonja Lyubomirsky (2007) and her colleagues found that participants practicing a similar gratitude exercise could increase their happiness over the course of 6 weeks, but, interestingly, this effect occurred only for individuals who did the exercise once a week (vs. three times a week), apparently because doing the exercise only weekly kept it fresh and meaningful.

This power of gratitude to boost well-being is recognized across cultures. In Japan, a particular form of psychotherapy called *Naikan* engages individuals in meditating on all the people who have cared for and helped them throughout their life. And the Vietnamese Buddhist monk Thich Nhat Hanh uses gratitude exercises to increase mindfulness, for example, calling attention to things we take for granted, such as the heart and its daily pumping of thousands of gallons of blood to nourish our bodies.

The power of gratitude extends to kids as well. In one study, 700 ten-year-old students filled out a gratitude questionnaire and then completed the questionnaire again at the end of 4 years ("Grateful teens," 2012). At the end of the 4-year period, the most grateful 20% had a 15% drop in negative emotions and had become 15%

more satisfied with their lives and 17% happier and more hopeful. The more grateful group was also slightly less likely to use alcohol and drugs, cheat on exams, and skip school.

About 4 years ago, when I first came across Lyubomirsky's work, I decided to do a gratitude exercise every day as a way to make myself more appreciative of what I have. Bob agreed to join me, and we eventually made it into a game with a couple of rules. Every day each of us names five things we are grateful for, and whoever is first to remember the exercise that day gets to go first, which is a little easier because whoever is second has to think of five *additional* things.

Although this exercise was difficult when we started, now both of us can easily reel off five new things to be grateful for per day. We've also noticed three unexpected positive effects that make it easier to remember and do. One, our gratitude is often for something the other one has done for us, and saying it aloud creates a positive feeling between us. Two, if one of us is getting bogged down in negativity, the other will suggest "let's do attitude of gratitude," and we do, which then usually shifts the person's negative focus. And three, when our religiously diverse family and friends get together for dinner, before eating we go around the table and everyone says one thing that they are grateful for—a form of blessing that creates a warm feeling and calls our attention to the variety of things for which we should all be grateful.

If you want to make this exercise a regular part of your life, the trick is to keep it interesting by adapting it in a way that works for you. Some people I've worked with use it in their morning devotions, others like to write their list in a journal, and some prefer to use it as a nightly mental ritual in bed before falling asleep. However you use it, because gratitude seems to be incompatible with irritation and anger, the exercise can help you let go of these unwanted emotions. In addition, you will start noticing things you take for granted, for example, that your partner told a friend something nice about you; or that when a stoplight went out, drivers respectfully took turns; or that the people who made your medications were careful to put the right ingredients in them. This increased mindfulness of the goodness around you is a well-being booster that positively affects the well-being of those around you too.

Try This: Attitude of Gratitude

A. Name five things you are deeply grateful for:
1. _____
2. _____
3. _____
4. _____
5. _____

Do you notice a positive feeling as you focus on these five things?

B. Continue to write or say aloud five new gratitudes every day for 1 week. Watch for a difference in how you feel at the time you make your list and throughout the week.

---

2. REFRAMING

Reframing is a form of countering in which you intentionally take a different perspective. You've probably experienced such a shift in perspective unintentionally, for example, when you complain about your demanding job and a kind coworker offers to help you, and then you learn that she is working three part-time jobs just to make ends meet. Or you're feeling angry about a minor health problem, then someone you care about is diagnosed with a life-threatening disease and doesn't have health insurance. Such shifts in perspective involve thoughts such as *Maybe I'm not that bad off,* followed by feelings of relief, gratitude, and compassion toward the other person—all of which feel much better than irritation, frustration, anxiety, or anger.

Reframing is a tool that enables you to deliberately create these positive feelings in spite of stressors that cannot be changed. It also calls your attention to positives in a given situation, opening the way for solutions you may have overlooked. In its simplest form, reframing involves asking yourself, *Is there another way to think about this problem that would help me feel less stressed?*

Reframing that specifically counters a stress-generating thought is usually the most helpful, for example:

> **Thought stressor:** *I can't stand that I have this diagnosis and the [health] problems that go along with it. Why me? It's not fair . . .*
>
> **Reframe:** *I don't like having this [medical problem], but it has given me more empathy for others, and brought some wonderful people into my life.*

Compassion voice (toward yourself or others) is often a type of reframe. For example, I once worked with a post office employee who had a difficult home life and was reaching the limits of his coping abilities during the Christmas season with the increase in impatient, angry customers. Previously, he'd told me about a recent trip to San Francisco and a person living on the street who yelled and called him names as he was walking by. When I asked why the San Francisco guy's behavior didn't bother him, he said, "I just thought of the guy as mentally ill and felt sorry for him." At my suggestion, he began applying this idea at work. In response to angry customers, instead of thinking *what a #$@%^*, which would increase *his* anger, he would say to himself: *If they're this upset about waiting 10 minutes to send* *a package during a time that's supposed to be about goodwill and cheer, they must have some impairment or a really sad life.*

3. WISE ELDER

One of my favorite thought-change tools is called *wise elder* (Dolan, 1991). One version of the wise elder is in the box below.

Try This: Wise Elder

1. Think of an external stressor that brings up negative thoughts and feelings of internally generated stress:_____
2. Now close your eyes and imagine that you are 90 years old, with a lifetime of experiences, learning, and wisdom. When you have a picture of yourself at this older age, go to the next step.
3. Now, as your 90-year-old self, imagine that you are looking back on this external stressor and your reaction to it. What advice would you give yourself? _____

_____

Do you notice a shift in your feelings as you tell yourself this advice?

A variation of wise elder is to think of someone you admire and respect. They can be living, deceased, a character in a book, or a religious figure. Ask yourself, *What would they do in this situation?* Then use this response as a guide. If your role model is someone you know well, you are probably aware of the person's weaknesses. However, if you've never met the person, be cautious about comparing yourself to a role model whom you perceive as perfect because this will probably not help you feel better.

On the other hand, if you are religiously inclined and believe in a compassionate, loving God, a similar type of reframe is to imagine how God would view your situation and what She/He would say to you or encourage you to do or not do. This works particularly well if some of your stress is coming from harsh, condemning thoughts about yourself or someone else.

4. GROWTH OPPORTUNITY

If these specific reframes are too difficult or do not fit your particular situation, Buddhists have a general one that works for everything, summarized in the saying *All obstacles are opportunities for growth*. Opportunities for growth include experiences that enable you to deepen your understanding of yourself and others, build new skills, and strengthen your self-confidence—in short, become a better person. With this reframe, obstacles are seen as a normal part of life, to be expected and handled as compassionately as possible with no need for the negative, judgmental thinking and behavior that make them more difficult.

The growth opportunity reframe involves asking yourself what you can learn and how you can grow from this experience, including a different outlook, greater empathy, more appreciation for what you have, and so on. It also involves considering how you want to behave in the face of this stressor.

Carol found the growth opportunity reframe especially helpful because it fit with her spiritual beliefs. Looking back on her life, she could see not only how growing up as an oldest child in a neglectful home was hard on her but also how it had contributed to her sense of purpose and internal strength. Although it seemed more difficult for her to see her *current* stressors as opportunities for growth, she decided to try. When she felt pressured by the demands on her time, she would remind herself that she didn't have to figure out a perfect balance and that working and caring for her family and friends *and* learning to pay attention to her own needs was a challenge. However, she had been through harder things before and knew that with her faith she could get through this and that she would come out in a better place.

Try This: Growth Opportunity

1. Think of an obstacle you faced in the past, which you worked through or resolved. Do you see any positive effects of this experience on your character, perspective, or life now?_____

   _____

2. Think of a current external stressor that brings up unwanted feelings in you, and ask yourself these Growth Opportunity questions.
   - What does my physical and emotional response to this stressor tell me about myself, my needs, my weak areas, and my strengths?

     _____

     _____

   - Is there something I can learn from this experience? _____

     _____

   - Even if there is no solution, how do I want to behave in the face of this? _____

     _____

   - Can I see how getting through this will make me a stronger, more understanding, or more patient person? _____

     _____

The preceding four tools—attitude of gratitude, reframing, wise elder, and growth opportunity—involve directly changing your thoughts. In contrast, these next two approaches are a little different in that they focus on increasing acceptance of your thoughts—even the highly distressing ones. These two tools change your relationship to your thoughts, which eventually will change your thinking too, and they are particularly helpful for internally generated stress that is especially resistant to change.

5. VALUES COMPASS

When you have tried and tried to change something in yourself, and either the change is not happening or it is going so slowly that you are getting discouraged, it can help to imagine your value priorities as an internal compass that keeps you motivated along the path of well-being. This approach works well when you are so focused on a problem behavior or character flaw that you believe nothing short of completely stopping, changing, or eliminating your shortcoming will help you feel better. With this tool, you do not ignore your own contribution to your stress; rather, you focus on the values that give you a sense of purpose as a way to motivate yourself to keep going when the going is tough.

Using your compassion voice to increase your acceptance, you encourage yourself with these kinds of thoughts: *OK, apparently I am not able to change this, at least for now, so I need to accept myself the way I am, the situation for what it is, or this person for who he or she is—at least for now. How can I live my life and make good choices despite this difficulty, in a way that fits with my values?*

This is a tough mental shift to make, but in an amazing paradox, the "acceptance of what is" usually eliminates the resistance and struggle that makes the change so difficult. As a result, later on the desired change often occurs, or alternative solutions become apparent that make the change easier.[1] It's like when you are trying to pull a tight ring off a swollen finger, and the harder you pull, the more the finger swells and holds the ring in place. When you give up and focus on something else instead, over time the swelling goes down and the ring comes off with little effort.

---

[1]There is a form of psychotherapy that focuses primarily on this concept of accepting what is and living according to your values. It is called *acceptance and commitment therapy*, and its originator is Steven Hayes.

For example, Marisol had struggled with a weight problem most of her life. She'd tried a variety of diets and exercise, and as a result, she had experienced periods of up to 2 years of eating well, exercising regularly, and maintaining a healthy weight. However, in the midst of too many external stressors, she would eventually "fall off the wagon" and became trapped in self-berating thoughts that sapped her energy to make even small changes.

As Marisol considered how changing her thinking might help, she decided to reframe her view of "my weight problem" to a positive focus on increasing her health. With this shift, even small steps such as not eating desserts or walking to the post office once a week made sense and helped her build a sense of progress.

Then, to motivate herself further, she returned to thinking about her values and remembered that her top priority was *peace*. She thought about what peace would mean and look like from every angle: peaceful interactions with her partner, daughters, and coworkers; feeling peaceful in the car during her long commute; and even being at peace with her weight. Her attention to the latter led to her recognition of thoughts that were undermining her sense of internal peace: *I can't stand to be this heavy, I hate the way I look, I absolutely have to lose this weight.* She began countering and replacing these thoughts stressors with

> OK, you don't like your weight, but it's not the end of the world that you are overweight, and it doesn't seem to bother anyone but you. And the fact is, you *can* stand it because you've had this difficulty for years. So give yourself some peace about this—just accept that you'll be this weight for a while longer, which is not forever, and focus instead on the small steps you need to get healthy physically and mentally. Keep remembering the sense of peace you give yourself during your walk in the woods, when you're not criticizing yourself at all, and how every little step you take toward being healthy helps your sense of peace grow.

Another way to approach this exercise is to think of your top value and then ask yourself, *What would a person who lives and shows this value do in this situation?* For example, if courage is one of your values, ask yourself, *What would a courageous person think, feel, and do in this situation?* A helpful response might be to tell yourself that even courageous people feel afraid; they just go ahead and do what they need to do anyway. As the saying goes: Courage is fear that has said its prayers.

Try This

1. Return to the Values Priority list you created in Chapter 1, and pick one of your top values:_____.
2. Name an external stressor that brings up stress in you: _____
   _____.
3. Ask yourself, *In response to this stressor or situation, what would a [insert value here]_____ person do?* _____
   _____
   _____.
4. Write a thought that motivates you by focusing on your value: _____
   _____

---

6. MEDITATION

Meditation is so effective in improving well-being that a leading magazine for psychologists recently explored its use in a special issue titled "Do We Even Need Any Psychotherapy Anymore?" (Simon, 2011). The authors concluded that there is a place for both, and many psychologists (including myself) incorporate meditation and mindfulness practices into psychotherapy.

There are many kinds of meditation: sitting meditation, walking meditation, loving kindness meditation, and yoga, to name a few. All of these various forms begin with attention to the breath. Breath is a tool in itself that connects your mind with your body. When you focus on your breath, you create a bridge that allows your mind to listen to your body, creating a *one-ness* of body and mind (Nhat Hanh, 1976).

Remember the mindfulness and focusing exercises you did in Chapter 4? Focusing on your breath in this intentional way allows you to observe your thoughts and feelings from a slight distance, which usually has a calming effect. You begin to recognize that you are not your thoughts or feelings, that your thoughts and feelings come and go, and that you can watch them come and go without being pulled into the thoughts or overwhelmed by the emotion. As meditation teacher Jon Kabat-Zinn (1994) says, "You can't stop the waves, but you can learn to surf" (p. 30).

If meditation is new to you, keep in mind that as you are trying to focus on your breath, it is completely normal for thoughts to intrude on your attempts. The goal is not to eliminate or change these thoughts or the related emotions. Rather, meditation is an exercise in *noticing* the thoughts and feelings, acknowledging and accepting that they are simply thoughts and feelings, then gently pulling your attention back to your breath, over and over, without judgment. If you remember that meditation is always just a practice, there is no need for judgment because there is no goal.

Try the meditation in the box above. In using this meditation exercise, I recommend starting small—5 minutes a day is fine for beginners. Then you can increase the time as you are able. If you want to do a longer meditation, psychologist Ron Siegel has a website that lists 16 different kinds of meditation you can download for your personal use, including *loving kindness, stepping into fear, urge surfing for pain, listening,* and *befriending the changes*.[2]

---

[2]http://www.mindfulness-solution.com

Try This: Mountain Meditation

Begin the same way you began the previous mindfulness exercises, sitting or lying comfortably with your eyes closed or gaze lowered, turning your attention to your breath. As you focus on your breath, notice the feeling of the air moving in through your nostrils and the air moving out through your nostrils. You may notice your attention being pulled away by noises around you, thoughts that pop into your head, or feelings that well up. If this happens, gently pull your attention back to your breath without any judgment about the distractions or about yourself. Continue to focus on the breath moving in, and the breath moving out, for a few minutes. Think of yourself as a mountain, sitting serenely, solidly grounded in the earth. Clouds swirl around you (like thoughts and feelings come and go through your head), but as the weather continually changes around you, none of it affects you, the mountain, as you continue to focus on your breath.

When you are ready to end the meditation, slowly bring your attention back into the room, wiggling your fingers and toes a little, and slowly open your eyes.

SMALL STEP

Choose one of the six well-being boosters—attitude of gratitude, reframing, wise elder, growth opportunity, values compass, or meditation—that sounds the easiest to you. During the next week, practice the exercise at least once a day and watch for effects on your thinking, emotions, body, and behavior.

Step 4:

TAKING ACTION

CHAPTER 10

THE POWER OF THOUGHT
AND ACTION

You miss 100% of the shots you never take.
> —Wayne Gretzky

Changing what and how you think can help you feel better, but when you combine the thought-change tools with action, you take charge of your life. In this chapter, we'll look at five action domains aimed at changing your environment and your behavior in ways that build well-being.

One cool, crisp September afternoon, as I headed out to the cranberry patch near our house (in Alaska), my mind was filled with thoughts of gratitude for the beautiful day, and my mood was equally positive. But then I saw a fresh pile of bear poop next to paw prints bigger than my boot. In response to the adrenaline rush (physical sensation) and feeling of fear (emotion), my thoughts suddenly shifted from gratitude to: *Oh crap, now I have to deal with this! I hate this—I can't even go out my front door without worrying about a bear attack.* Terrifying images started to pop into my mind, and then I launched into the most effective countering I could muster: *OK, you know, bears are more afraid of people than you are of them; they're really shy; you've seen plenty, and in every case, they ran away as fast as they could, and there have never been any bear attacks on our road, at least not on people.*

But despite my best mental efforts, a persistent, low-level anxiety threatened to ruin my favorite autumn activity—that is, until I admitted to myself that trying to change my thinking was not enough. Recognizing the need for some action, I headed back to the house, got a can of bear spray from the garage, and returned to the berry patch. With the bear spray in hand, my anxiety subsided, my thoughts turned back to an appreciation of the beautiful day, and I continued picking berries until my bucket was full.

Up until now, we've focused on decreasing stress with thought-change tools, whether the source of your stress is an external stressor or your own thinking. But as with my bear fears, sometimes thought-change is not enough, or it's clear that taking action will help you feel better more quickly and efficiently.

As I mentioned earlier, I started with the thought-change tools primarily for organizational purposes. But often the most effective way to feel better and build well-being involves a combination of thought change *and* action. So now in Step 4, we'll focus more on action, including changing your environment and changing your behavior.

WHERE TO START?

Because thoughts, feelings, and behavior are so intertwined, and all occur within the same environment, any change in one usually leads to a change in the other. That is, if you change something in your environment, you will probably notice changes in your thoughts, feelings, and behavior. Sometimes your new thoughts, feelings, and behavior even affect your environment. For example, when you are feeling blue but smile at people anyway, they smile back and you feel a little better, which makes it easier to keep smiling, which brings you more smiles from others.

So where's the best place to start: changing your thinking, your behavior, or your environment? One approach is to start with whatever is easiest for you, and if that doesn't work, then to try another. For example, in response to the bear scat, I tried thinking differently first because it took less physical effort, but my anxiety did not decrease, so then I took action. My action simultaneously involved a change in my behavior (taking the bear spray with me) and a change to my environment (adding a safety item). This action helped me feel better and facilitated more helpful thinking, which in this case included a realistic recognition of possible danger without obsessing about it.

From the beginning, Marisol recognized that to become healthier and bring more peace into her life, she would need to make changes in her behavior and in her work and home environments. But she didn't have much hope that her actions would make a difference because she'd already tried so many things that didn't work—a variety of diets, skipping meals, buying too-tight pants to inspire herself to lose weight, and paying for a gym membership she rarely used.

All of these failed attempts increased her self-berating thoughts, which made her feel worse about herself and further decreased her energy to take action. So she decided to start this time by becoming more accepting of herself with kinder, gentler self-talk. As she increased attention to her strengths and values and shifted her desire to lose weight to the goal of increasing her health, she experienced greater optimism about trying new things and more energy to take action. For example, she began recognizing that easier access to unhealthy foods influenced her food choices at home and work, that she controlled a great deal of the food coming into her house because she did most of the grocery shopping, and that she could choose what she kept in her desk at work for snacks. She also noticed that, for one of her coworkers, socializing consisted mostly of physical activities—biking, hiking, lunch-hour walking, playing games with friends—which contrasted sharply with her own assumption that socializing had to involve eating.

In contrast, for Sheldon, taking action was more in his comfort zone than paying attention to his thinking. Right after his girlfriend left, he was not ready to look at his own part in his emotional pain (which is what changing one's thinking involves), so instead he changed his physical and social environment one night per week by going to the basketball court. This first small action step created positive feelings that over time opened him to thinking about how his attitude, self-talk, and behavior might be working against him.

Carol, on the other hand, recognized right away that she wanted to feel better about herself and that this would involve being less judgmental and letting go of the belief that she constantly needed to take care of others. Her subsequent reframing of her needs as important and her increased focus on her strengths and supports built her optimism that she could be happier. However, she continued to have painful interactions with her husband and daughter because she still needed to learn how to be more assertive and follow through with better self-care, a vital part of well-being that is covered in Chapter 13.

WHAT ACTION?

When you are feeling overwhelmed by negative emotions, it can be as difficult to see what action might help as it is to see how your thinking is the problem. So as a reminder of the range of actions that decrease stress and build well-being, I use an acronym that spells the word *CLASS*. *C* stands for *Create a healthy environment*—one that facilitates good choices and helpful behavior. *L* stands for *Learn and practice well-being behavior* such as meditation, a hobby you enjoy, or a new way of doing something that helps you meet your long-term goals. Well-being behaviors also include *Assertiveness, conflict resolution, and other communication skills* that improve your relationships; *Social engagement* that brings with it practical help from others, emotional support, and a sense of meaning and purpose; and *Self-care* activities that build your physical, mental, and spiritual strength to tackle problems that are solvable and accept those that are not.

There is often some overlap between these areas. For example, increasing your social engagement requires *behavioral* changes that also change your social *environment*. Whether you focus on the behavioral or environmental changes involved with action steps, the important point is to recognize that an action step is often necessary, easier, or more effective than thought change alone.

In some situations, action steps can eliminate or minimize a stressor directly—for example, when Marisol began taking her family out to dinner on soccer nights to eliminate the stressor of cooking. But even when a stressor cannot be changed, an action step may buffer the effects of the stressor so that you don't experience so much stress. Although Sheldon was still hurting about his girlfriend's departure and feeling the pressure of work, each time he went out with his coworkers he created a more positive feeling toward them that made his work a little easier that week.

CLASS Actions That Counter Stress and Build Well-Being

- **C**reate a healthy environment;
- **L**earn and practice well-being behavior, including:
- **A**ssertiveness, conflict resolution, and other communication skills;
- **S**ocial engagement; and
- **S**elf-care activities.

One final point regarding action is that most of the action steps you take, whether they involve environmental or behavioral change, are ones that will help you throughout your life. Just as you did with the thought-change tools, when you are ready to take action, remember the principle of small steps, because this will increase the likelihood you will stick with your positive actions even after the stress is gone.

In Chapter 11, we turn to the first of these action steps: creating a healthy environment.

CHAPTER 11

CREATE A HEALTHY ENVIRONMENT

The environment is everything that isn't me.

—Albert Einstein

Because our environments strongly influence what we think, feel, and do, a good place to begin taking action is with our immediate surroundings. By creating a healthy environment, you can shape and influence your thoughts, feelings, and behavior in ways that improve your physical and psychological well-being.

When I talk about making environmental change, people often think of big changes like moving to another state, going back to school, or looking for a new job. Although such changes definitely affect a person's mood and behavior, there are also many smaller changes you can make to your daily environment that facilitate good choices and healthy behavior. These environmental changes may target a specific behavior that you want to increase or decrease, or they may be aimed at improving your general well-being. Let's start with the first: environmental influences on specific behaviors.

SHAPING SPECIFIC BEHAVIORS

Psychologists have long known that behavior can be created, shaped, and even eliminated through environmental interventions. For example, arranging classroom chairs in a circle facilitates class discussions, whereas lining up desks in rows does not. At home, the arrangement of rooms and furniture subtly influences how, where, and when people interact, as do public spaces and building architecture on a larger scale.

If you are trying to change a specific behavior, it is important to pay attention to how the environment elicits and rewards the *undesired* behavior and to look for environmental changes you can make to encourage and reward the *desired* behavior. For example, as Marisol focused on making her environment healthier, she realized that having a "sweet treats" drawer at work made it too easy to eat a candy bar when her energy slumped at 4 p.m. As she became more aware of the greater accessibility of unhealthy snacks than of healthy foods at her workplace and in her home, she took small, gradual steps to change what she could. She couldn't stop coworkers from leaving food to share in the lunchroom, but she replaced her candy drawer with cut-up fruits and vegetables and stopped buying her favorite snack foods for home.

Over time, as she became more mindful of the influence of her environment on her eating habits, she began placing healthy foods in the refrigerator door where they were easier to grab, eating her meals off smaller plates, using smaller cups for drinks with calories, and so on. (I'll talk more about environmental factors and mindful eating in Chapter 15.)

Another small environmental change toward her goal of healthy, peaceful living was to stop listening to the news during her morning commute; instead, she played soothing music or listened to an inspirational CD. This small step positively affected her body via increased relaxation; her thoughts, through inspiring messages that she internalized and used as self-talk; and her emotions, which became more positive as a result.

Sheldon knew that his drinking wasn't helping him live a more fulfilling life. Recognizing that he drank more when he was home alone than when he was out with friends, he stopped buying alcohol for his house. This action had the added effect of saving him money, which loosened the hold of his repetitive thought that he shouldn't relax because he needed to save money. In this way, his action changed his thinking. His new thoughts (e.g., *If I don't take some time for fun, I'll burn myself out and I could lose my job and then I would really have money problems*) made it easier for him to put work aside and do something enjoyable.

Sheldon also recognized the pull of his home computer, which always contained work. It was too big a step to stop using the computer when he was home, so instead he chose to increase his time in an environment where his computer and work were not available. Specifically, he volunteered to coach a kids' intramural basketball team at the rec center, which required him to be there 3 nights a week. In addition to decreasing his drinking and home–work time on the computer, these steps had the added effect of increasing his social involvement. The positive social interactions and expressions of appreciation from parents were much more enjoyable than his drinking and excessive computer work had been, and so those behaviors gradually decreased. These environmental and behavioral changes increased his positive thoughts about others and helped him feel better.

Although I distinguish between environmental and behavioral changes with separate chapters in this book, the two often overlap, as the examples of Marisol and Sheldon show. Changing your environment invariably requires that you *do* something (i.e., act). But sometimes it's clearly your environment that needs to change. For example, if you work in a setting that supports racist or similarly oppressive behaviors, or if you live in an abusive home, *your* behavior is not the problem. This may seem obvious to some, but sometimes in situations like these, individuals begin to blame themselves and believe that if they just change some specific behaviors or thinking patterns, they can stop the abuse and all will be well. Simply put: There are some environments that no one should have to adapt to.

IMPROVING GENERAL WELL-BEING

Even if you do not have a specific behavior you want to change, you can still make changes in your environment that help you feel better and, over time, build well-being. Start by thinking about small actions that you might take to make your work space healthier, more comfortable, and helpful. If you do a lot of computer work, consider ergonomics—for example, the height of your desk, computer, and keyboard; the type of click your mouse or pointer requires; the posture your chair encourages. Most of the work done with computers does not create health problems, but using equipment incorrectly or too intensely can lead to repetitive stress injuries that take a long time to heal.

Also, think about the arrangement of furniture and equipment in a way that builds physical and mental breaks into your routine. For example, I know a woman who recently had back surgery. When she returned to work, she deliberately used the printer located in another room to force herself to get up from her desk and walk to the printer to pick up her document. Ironically, well-intentioned coworkers began bringing her documents to her, until she explained to them that she wanted to walk to the printer because these small exercise steps were important for her physical healing.

Consider your physical surroundings as a potential source of inspiration. Bring a little nature into your space with a potted plant that adds oxygen to the room or even fake flowers that add cheerful color. Put a beautiful, relaxing, or inspiring scene in your work space with a calendar or on your computer screen, and look at it mindfully to give yourself a brief mental break. Photos that bring up positive feelings may do the same thing. If calming background music does not interfere and helps you work, add some. One of the smallest steps I remember a client describing to me once was bringing a piece of velvet to her desk; she said it felt comforting to touch. You might program your computer to give you reminder beeps to take these little mental and physical breaks.

Sayings posted in your work space, car, or around the house can be used to remind you of your long-term goals, values, and purpose and help you reinforce positive self-talk. Alcoholics Anonymous has many great sayings: *One day at a time; Fake it till you make it; First things first; Do I want to be happy or be right?* Mothers are another good source of sayings, and I use the following one from my mom regarding frustrating situations: *Nothing lasts forever.* Another source of sayings are songs that have a message you like.

The Importance of Light

Sunshine also has a powerful effect on mood. For example, here in Alaska, during the winter when the sun is out for only a few hours, we sleep more and do less, and the incidence of depression increases. Exposure to outdoor light helps to counter seasonal affective disorder, which is probably why we have so many outdoor winter sports (skiing, snowshoeing, ice skating, ice fishing, winter walking, dog mushing, and snowmachining). One study at the University of Colorado found that only 30 minutes per day of being outdoors significantly improved mood (Walsh, 2011). Additional research has found that bright artificial light that mimics sunlight can have a similar effect, and one of the easiest ways to artificially obtain it is with a light therapy box (Mayo Clinic, 2013). (My sister swears that her light box works best when she eats a piece of cream-cheese frosted carrot cake while sitting in front of it.)

People vary in their sensitivity to light, and for some people, different types of light have different effects. Several of the counselors

I work with have replaced their overhead office fluorescents with desk lamps because they say the softer light feels calming (although to me it feels depressing). One other suggestion on the topic of lighting is that if you have a hard time waking up in the dark, consider buying a sunrise alarm clock. I set mine for 7:30 a.m., and the attached globe light comes on gradually beginning at 7 a.m. until it is fully lit; if my eyes are still closed, I have the sensation that sunlight is streaming into the room. As far as I know, this kind of light does not affect mood, but it makes it much easier way to wake up.

Sounds of Silence

Sound can be a low-level, unperceived stressor. For example, during the 3 years I lived in a high-rise apartment between a main highway and an exit ramp in downtown Honolulu, I mostly tuned out the constant roar of the highway and the loud stop-and-start of cars on the exit ramp. However, on visits home to Alaska, as I stepped off the small plane at our little airport, I would immediately experience the silence, which seemed to settle into my body and drain away the tension.

In fact, unwanted environmental sound (defined as noise) has been linked to heart disease, high blood pressure, gastrointestinal disorders, headaches, fatigue, insomnia, and poor concentration (Goud, 2001). But because we humans have such an amazing ability to adapt, we often don't perceive noise to be a stressor, particularly white (background) noise. Although some noise pollution is uncontrollable, there are actions you can take to minimize your exposure. But first it helps to become more mindful of the noise around you and its effects on your physical and emotional state.

Here are a few suggestions for changing your soundscapes in ways that decrease stress and, over time, build well-being (Goud,

---

Try This

Increase your awareness of the *soundscapes* in which you live by closing your eyes right now and naming all of the sounds you notice: _____
_____.

What are the physical sensations and emotions you notice as you listen to these sounds?_____.

Try this exercise in different locations, and pay attention to the feelings you experience in reaction to different soundscapes.

2001). As you try these, pay attention to your mental and physical reactions.

- Notice the sounds—including silence—that create a feeling of peace in you, and build them into your daily routine. If you are lucky enough to live close to nature, listen for the sounds of a trickling creek, the wind blowing softly, birds singing, or rain on the roof. If not, add a trickling fountain, soft wind chimes, or other soothing sound to your environment.
- Deliberately play music that brings you the positive feeling you want, such as relaxation, energy, joy, power, and peace.
- Treat yourself to a rest break in a quiet place, if possible, outdoors; for example, sit on a park bench or walk in the woods.
- Avoid masking sound with more sound (e.g., talking louder over the sound of the TV). Turn off the background noise.
- Know your sound limits, that is, the kinds of sounds that make you feel agitated or irritated.
- Unplug devices that ring or buzz, for example, your computer, cell phone, and overhead lights, at least for a period of time to give yourself a break.

Intellectual Stimulation

Learning is a necessary component of human growth and development. Healthy people are drawn to new experiences and new information. I've often wondered if the reason people look forward to traveling when they retire is because traveling brings so many opportunities for learning without performance expectations.

I'll talk more about the importance of learning new behavior as we move through the CLASS actions, but I mention it here to make the point that the opposite of learning and growth, boredom, can be a big stressor. And your environment is influential when it comes to opportunities for intellectual stimulation.

Now that her children were grown and her mother-in-law had died, part of Carol's problem was a lack of intellectual stimulation and opportunity to learn new things. When she was at the house all day (the house she'd lived in for 20 years), she felt depressed. She tried making changes to her house, including the addition of brighter lights, but they were not enough. Her depressed mood led her to turn down invitations from friends because she didn't want to burden them. The more she isolated herself, the more irritable she became. This increased her negative interactions with her husband, who was home most of the day because he was retired. When she felt low, she had even more difficulty saying no to her daughter's babysitting requests.

Initially Carol did not perceive her own behavior to be part of the problem; that is, she blamed her negative interactions on her husband's crabbiness and her daughter's unreasonable expectations. However, she *was* aware that she needed to make changes in her environment. So she took a big step, looking for and eventually finding a full-time job. Her decision to return to paid employment put her in a new environment with a variety of people, which enriched her life. She enjoyed and appreciated her free time more and was better able to tell her daughter *no* (although she still felt some guilt and needed to learn better communication skills). Because she was working in social services, her work fit nicely with the value she placed on helping others but required her to stop at 5 p.m. Like Sheldon, changing her environment enabled Carol to see how her thoughts, beliefs, and behavior might be contributing to her unhappiness (as described earlier in the thought-change chapters).

SMALL STEP

Keeping in mind all five senses, look for environmental influences that create a calm, positive feeling in you—for example, something you look at (a beautiful picture), listen to (music), smell (a scented candle), taste (chamomile tea), or physically feel (a comfy blanket). Alternatively, make a small change in your environment that facilitates a healthy choice or desired behavior. Throughout the week, watch for the effects of this small change on your thoughts, feelings, and behavior.

CHAPTER 12

LEARN AND PRACTICE WELL-BEING BEHAVIOR

We are what we practice, and we are always practicing something.
—Staci Haines[1]

In addition to creating a healthy environment, you can decrease stress and increase your well-being with specific behaviors. The Seven Behavior Change Rules will help you begin your positive behavior changes and ensure that these changes will last.

Well-being behaviors span a wide range and include easy ones that are enjoyable to do as well as challenging ones that require effort but pay off in the long run. Using the CLASS acronym (with **C** for Creating a healthy environment and **L** for Learning and practicing well-being behaviors), the well-being behaviors can be divided into three categories: (a) Assertiveness, conflict resolution, and other communication skills that make social interactions smoother and more rewarding; (b) Social engagement, which acts as a stress buffer and builds well-being in and around us; and (c) Self-care activities such as getting enough sleep, eating well, exercising, and fun activities that help you feel better.

---

[1]From the Therapeutic Justice Project blog, http://therapeuticjustice. blogspot.com/

We'll look at each of these three categories in the three chapters that follow this one, but first I want to share with you seven key principles that will help you with the *process* of learning, practicing, and maintaining your new behavior. These principles are taught in most first-year psychology programs. They are the core of many advice books, and they are central to what psychotherapists do with clients. I call them the *Seven Behavior Change Rules* because if you follow them, you ensure that your changes will last.

THE SEVEN BEHAVIOR CHANGE RULES

Rule 1. Ask Yourself What the Unwanted Behavior Does for You

This rule should sound familiar because it's one of the steps in self-compassion, in which you caringly seek to understand your behavior, including what you get from the unwanted behavior. Although the disadvantages of an unwanted behavior are usually obvious, it is often difficult to see the advantages. But we all engage in behaviors for a reason, even if the reason is long gone and the behavior continues out of habit. It is important to understand the reason for a behavior because if the behavior fills some need that will not get met when you change the behavior, then the change is not likely to stick.

Another way to think of this rule is that before you take something away, you need to put something positive in its place. Otherwise, there will be a vacuum where the old behavior or thought was, and we all know what a vacuum does—it sucks in the unwanted junk.

For example, Marisol recognized that there were many enjoyable aspects to her overeating. Most of her fun social relationships, happy family events, and leisure activities revolved around food. Food was also an easy source of comfort that did not bother others. She realized that her need for socialization and comfort were normal human needs that could not and should not be ignored and began to look for ways to socialize and comfort herself that did not involve food.

Sheldon was aware that his workaholic behavior earned him praise and respect from others and contributed to him having a job that paid well. What was less obvious to him, until he considered his behavior with compassion, was how his excessive work focus was connected to his childhood experiences of being teased. These early bullying experiences created a fear of rejection that increased his avoidance of social activities. He began to notice how often he used the excuse of "needing to work" to avoid new and awkward social situations and that this behavior worked against his desire to have a richer social life. He saw the helpfulness in replacing his automatic thought of *I have to get this done now* with compassionate self-talk that encouraged him to prioritize his social life.

Similarly, when Carol thought about the benefits of her excessive caretaking (even while neglecting her own needs), she could see a connection to her childhood fears of being abandoned. She remembered the positive part of taking care of her mother and siblings—a feeling of being needed—and recognized how this tendency influenced her relationships as an adult. She saw how continually doing more for another person than that person did for her ensured that the other person would need her and never leave. She realized that she could replace the fear-inducing thoughts with more realistic thoughts that helped her modify her helping behavior and pay attention to her own needs and desires too.

Rule 2. Frame Change as Increasing the Positive Rather Than Decreasing the Negative

Framing your change in positive terms keeps you focused on the positive. In addition, it is often easier to *start* doing a positive behavior than to *stop* doing a negative behavior. This is true for thoughts as well. For example, if I tell you to not think about a pink elephant, you are now thinking about a pink elephant. Even as you tell yourself *Stop thinking about that pink elephant!* you are thinking about it because you have to, in order to think *Don't think about it.* But if I tell you to think about a purple giraffe instead, it is easier to focus your mind on the purple giraffe, and the purple giraffe thought then replaces the pink-elephant-not-thought.[2] In this way, the more you focus on adding a new positive behavior or thought, the less opportunity there is to engage in the old negative one, until eventually the negative one drops out or becomes much less attractive.

Here are some examples of how Marisol, Sheldon, and Carol thought about their desired behavior changes in negative terms, then with their positive reframes.

Marisol
Negative: *Lose weight.*
Positive reframe: *Improve my physical, mental, and spiritual health.*

Sheldon
Negative: *Stop working so much.*
Positive reframe: *Enjoy my life more, have more friends, a comfortable home, and eventually get married.*

Carol
Negative: *Stop blowing up at people.*
Positive reframe: *Increase positive interactions with others.*

---

[2]Idea from Wegner (2011).

Rule 3. Set SMART Goals

Simply *setting* a goal increases the likelihood of sticking with a change. In a recent study conducted at the University of Scranton, researchers found that people who made a formal New Year's resolution were 10 times more likely to change than those with identical goals and comparable motivation who did not make formal resolutions (Norcross, Mrykalo, & Blagys, 2002).

SMART goals were first described in the field of business management but can be applied to any goals that involve behavioral change.[3] SMART goals are Specific, Measurable, Achievable, Relevant, and Time sensitive.

Specific, measurable, time-sensitive goals will help you assess your progress because you can see the results in numerical terms. Looking at the number, size, frequency and/or duration of your new behavior tells you in a concrete way whether your approach is working. You can also use this data to counter self-defeating thoughts when your progress slows. For example, in response to automatic thoughts of *What's the use? I might as well give up,* you can remind yourself and see that you *are* making progress compared with when you started. In the box below, I have provided some examples of vague goals translated into specific, measurable, and positive terms.

SMART goals are Achievable, meaning they are realistic given your particular capabilities, time frame, and internal and external resources. They are also Relevant to your values, aspirations, and current life. One of the mistakes people commonly make is setting a goal that is not humanly possible, for example, eliminating anger, never craving anything, or stopping all negative thinking. Such perfectionistic goals are called the *dead man's solution,* because only a

---

[3]The first known use of this acronym was in an article by George T. Doran (1981).

Example SMART Goals

Vague Goal →	Specific, Measurable, Time-sensitive, & Positive Goal
Be friendlier	Say hello to at least two people per day
Eat healthier	Breakfast of oatmeal, fruit, nonfat milk 6 days per week
Exercise more	Attend one exercise class per week
Be less critical	Compliment or thank someone at least once per day
Be calmer	Do one 10-minute relaxation exercise per day
Be less depressed	Plan and do one enjoyable activity per day

---

dead man never gets angry, never craves anything, and never makes a mistake.

If you are unsure whether your goal is achievable, ask two people who will tell you honestly. Then begin with the *small steps* approach. If it is easier to think of your long-term goal, go ahead and start with it, but then break it down into smaller, short-term goals and corresponding small steps. To make sure that each will move you toward your goal and be completely doable, ask yourself, *How sure am I that I can and will do this step—60% sure, 80% sure, or 100% sure?*" If you are not 100% sure, then make the step smaller. And when choosing the next step, follow the path of least resistance. Even a tiny first step begins a snowball of positives.

Toward the broader positive goal of improving her health, one of Marisol's SMART goals was to eat a healthy snack in place of an unhealthy one at 4 p.m., at least 6 days per week. This goal was relevant to her health and to her desire to feel better about herself and lose weight. She made it achievable by allowing for the one-day exception.

Sheldon's goal was to socialize and enjoy life more, which he decided to try at work, in addition to his after work activities.

The smallest step he could think of was to go out to lunch with a coworker, friend, or family member at least once a week. He figured that once a week was doable, but trying to go more often would have the opposite effect of increasing his pressured feeling.

In order to improve her positive interactions with others, Carol set a SMART goal of increasing her self-care by taking one hour of "me-time" per day. This goal was relevant to her need for better self-care, which helped her feel calmer and less irritated with others. She made her goal achievable by counting a broad range of behaviors as me-time, for example, taking a hot bath, reading a novel, having decompression time alone in her room after work, quilting, or whatever helped her feel better and fit with her values and long-range goal of improving her relationships.

Rule 4. Increase Facilitators and Minimize Obstacles

Facilitators are situations, events, people, timing, and anything else that helps you follow through with your goals. *Obstacles* are the opposite—anything that works against you reaching your goals. Both are person specific. That is, joining a class may be a facilitator for one person who wants to exercise more, but an obstacle for another person who has to find a babysitter and transportation and schedule extra travel time to and from the class. Having exercise equipment at home might be a big facilitator for this second person, but not at all for the first person, who likes the structured time and socializing that come with a class.

Once you recognize the facilitators and obstacles for your particular goal, increasing the former and minimizing the latter will greatly increase your chances of success. For example, keeping her drawers stocked with healthy foods was a facilitator for Marisol to eat a healthy snack instead of an unhealthy one. The ever-present plate of cookies in the lunchroom was an obstacle that she could not eliminate, so to minimize its influence, she used helpful self-talk, and at her low willpower time of 4 p.m., ate her healthy snack to increase her energy before going into the lunchroom for a break. (More on increasing willpower in Chapter 15.)

Telling others about your goal can be a facilitator if it brings you support and/or creates a greater feeling of accountability. Sheldon used this approach, telling his supervisor of his commitment to the kids' basketball team and that he would need to leave on time at 5 p.m. 3 nights each week. His supervisor was supportive and even helped him restructure his workload in advance. One obstacle was the flurry of last-minute e-mails that often arrived between 4 and 5 p.m., so Sheldon told his coworkers and the people he supervised that they could send him e-mails between 4 and 5 p.m. but not to expect a response until the next day.

To facilitate her daily self-care activity, Carol took a few minutes Sunday afternoon to schedule her 1 hour of me-time in her appointment book for the entire week. An obstacle was her varied schedule during and after work; for example, sometimes she had an hour for lunch that she could use, but not always, and sometimes she had errands to run after work that prevented her from taking me-time right after work. To minimize this obstacle of unpredictability, she did not try to stick with the same time every day, but rather scheduled her 1 hour around the demands of each day.

Rule 5. Reinforce the Behavior You Want to Increase

Behavior lasts because it is reinforced. This applies to good behavior and bad behavior, to adults and children. Furthermore, reinforcement works better than punishment. This is why child development experts emphasize giving kids lots of positive reinforcement for good behavior; kids need attention, and if they don't get it for good behaviors, they'll engage in bad behaviors to get the attention, even if the attention is punishing.

One easy way to reinforce a desired behavior is to pair it with a high-frequency behavior. For example, if you are trying to remember to read your Personal Strengths Inventory daily, put it on the bathroom mirror, so you will be reminded to read it every time you brush your teeth.

Another approach is to reinforce the performance of your desired behavior with something that makes you feel good. This includes encouraging, helpful self-talk and tangible rewards. Both are important, especially when the new behavior takes willpower to do (e.g., beginning to exercise, eat healthy foods, or go to bed on time).

To maximize the effect of a reward, it helps to match the size and cost of a reward to the size and effort of your step or goal. For example, if you are trying to exercise daily, you probably would not reward yourself for your first day of exercise by buying yourself a new outfit. A more reasonable (and affordable) reward might be a low-fat latté right after you exercise, a new book or magazine after a week of consistent exercise, then maybe the new outfit after a month or two.

Rewards are person specific, so you are the judge of what will reinforce your new behavior. There are some ideas to get you started in the box on the next page. With your own list, try to include some reinforcers that don't cost anything, because this eliminates the obstacle of money.

Rule 6. Track Your Progress

If you are trying to change a behavior and are unsure of a first small step, one of the smallest steps you can take is to simply pay attention to the behavior and record each time it occurs, including the

---

Try This

Circle the following items that would be reinforcers for you. Then add additional ones you can think of.

reading a favorite magazine
downloading a new app
watching a funny YouTube video, movie, or TV show
eating a favorite food
taking a relaxing bath
reading a good book
beading, sewing, or other craft
skiing, hiking, or other outdoor activity
e-mailing or phoning a friend
buying something new to wear
woodworking
trying out a new recipe
planning a road or camping trip
cooking or baking a favorite food
a walk on the beach
painting, drawing, listening to or playing music
others:

_____

_____

_____

---

situational specifics and your reaction. For example, if you're trying to stop smoking, you could keep a log of every time you smoke a cigarette, including the time of day, where you are, who you're with, and what you're doing. You can also do this with thoughts, for example, recording on your smartphone every time you intentionally think a positive thought within a specified period of time and what is going on at the time, including the time of day, where you are, who you're with, and what you're doing. Keeping track of your behavior provides a reminder of your improvements during times when you're feeling discouraged, and it can give you helpful information regarding facilitators and obstacles along your path.

There is something magical in the way that paying attention to a behavior leads to desired behavior change—a phenomenon known as the *Hawthorne effect.* During the 1920s, researchers at the Hawthorne Works Electric Plant began monitoring the effects of light intensity on workers' performance and found that productivity improved when the office light was increased. However, they subsequently found that productivity also improved when the office light was dimmed. It turned out (and subsequent studies confirmed) that simply paying attention to the workers' behavior created an expectation of positive change (i.e., improved performance) that resulted in improved performance. A related phenomenon is the *self-fulfilling prophecy,* in which a person looks for a specific behavioral outcome and finds it because the person's expectation influences his or her own or the other person's behavior. This is why when you're trying to lose weight and begin by tracking what you eat in a food journal, you usually eat less.

To track her healthy behaviors, Marisol used a calendar that showed 1 month at a time and wrote the specific healthy behaviors she did in the spot for each day. For example, under Monday, April 5, she wrote "30 min. walk @ lunch, healthy 4 p.m. snack," and then under Tuesday, April 6, "30 min. inspirational CD, healthy 4 p.m. snack."

Sheldon decided to keep track of the number of hours he spent doing fun social activities. He recorded the time each day on his smartphone, which gave him a total at the end of the week and month. He liked the positive feeling he experienced when he compared his starting point of 2 hours per week with his more recent higher number.

To track her progress on self-care, Carol put a check mark next to every day in her appointment book when she took her me-time. Because her me-time was part of her larger goal of improving her relationships, she also tracked her progress with social interactions. For this, she used a format developed by cognitive therapists called the Thought Record (Beck, Wright, Newman, & Liese, 1993). She began by recording twice a day—once when she felt a sense of well-being or at least felt calmer and once when she felt irritated—her feelings, the situation (what was going on, who was there, where, and when), her behavior, and thoughts at the time. Carol's Thought Record is in the box below.

Carol's Thought Record

Negative interaction:

- Feelings (emotion and physical sensation)—*irritated, tense*
- Situation—*in a hurry in the morning, went to the fridge and saw there was no milk for my cereal.*
- Thoughts—*Sal drank the milk last night and never bothered to tell me. He just expects me to keep the fridge stocked because I always have. He completely takes me for granted.*
- Behavior—*snapped at Sal and left for work without saying goodbye.*

Positive interaction:

- Feelings (emotion and physical sensations)—*happy, optimistic, relaxed*
- Situation—*at first I came home late, tired, and hungry, but Sal seemed glad to see me and had a nice dinner ready for me.*
- Thoughts—*OK, he's trying. I know he really loves me. He just wants to spend more time with me.*
- Behavior—*I hugged and thanked him, and interacted warmly, even when he made a comment about my work taking so much time.*

Using the Thought Record, Carol became more aware of her part in negative interactions with her husband. She began to notice how, if she was thinking positively about him, she felt kinder toward him, and these positive thoughts and feelings then affected her behavior positively. Specifically, she was less reactive to comments he made that would normally set her off. She became more aware of her own power to influence an interaction rather than blaming him for a negative one, and this awareness helped her with her other relationships too.

One thing to note if you want to use the Thought Record yourself is that you can vary the order of the categories depending on what works for you. Carol usually noticed her physical sensations and emotions first, so she started with that and then went on to describe the situation, her thoughts, and behavior. However, if your behavior is the first thing that you usually notice in yourself, you can start with that and then continue on by describing your feelings and thoughts. Do what works for you.

Rule 7. Consider Every Change You Make as an Experiment and Anticipate Setbacks

Scientists do not expect to find what they're looking for the first time they do an experiment; the research process takes time, and breakthroughs are usually accomplished after many failed attempts. But these failures continually push the research forward, ruling out what doesn't work, honing in on what will.

Similarly, when you want to change a behavior, it is helpful to think of your efforts as an experiment. If your first step doesn't work, think about the possible reasons in a helpful, caring way. Ask yourself these questions:

- Is my long-range goal realistic?
- Was my step too big?
- Do I need to break this step down into smaller steps?
- Was there an obstacle I did not anticipate?
- Did I overlook a possible facilitator?

When you're trying to change, it is important to recognize that you will not do it perfectly, nor will your physical and social environment respond perfectly to the changes you make in yourself. Anticipating setbacks helps you decrease the surprises when they happen and plan for how you can get yourself back on track as quickly as possible.

Marisol knew from years of dieting that when she overate, the thought *Well, I've already blown it, so I might as well give it up* led her to continue to overeat for the rest of the day, which made it even more difficult to get back on track the following day. Anticipating that she would still have times of overeating, or eating the wrong thing, she practiced in advance what she would say to herself: *OK, I messed up, but I can get back on track with my next meal (or the next day)*. In addition, her healthy environmental changes made it easier to stick with her behavioral changes.

Sheldon recognized that he would still have times when work would build up and there would be negative consequences for not getting it done right away. This is why he still kept 2 nights a week and parts of his weekend open—just in case.

Carol knew that although she could increasingly control her own behavior, sometimes other people's behavior would affect her and create changes beyond her control. For example, if she or her husband developed a serious health problem (which many of their peers had), she might not be able to keep up her current schedule. She began to think ahead about this and how she could still meet her needs for intellectual stimulation and positive social engagement if she were to work part time.

SMALL STEP

Think of a behavior you would like to change and create a relevant SMART goal for yourself.

Name the specific behavior you want to increase or decrease
_____

How can you measure it?_____

How can you make it achievable and realistic?_____
_____

Is it relevant to your values and life goals?_____

What is your time frame? _____

Name at least one facilitator _____
_____

Name at least one obstacle and how you will minimize it_____
_____

Name at least one reinforcer _____
_____

CHAPTER 13

ASSERTIVENESS, CONFLICT RESOLUTION, AND OTHER COMMUNICATION SKILLS

Communication works for those who work at it.
—John Powell

Healthy relationships are central to well-being. Healthy relationships depend on respectful communication that keeps you connected, even when you disagree.

One day after I'd been in clinical practice for several years, it suddenly occurred to me that every person I'd seen that week was coming in for a relationship problem—an angry couple on the verge of divorce, a parent and teen ready to disown each other, an adult child concerned about their aging parent, and so on. I looked at my calendar of appointments for that month and saw that nearly every one involved a relationship issue. Even those few that did not primarily concern relationships (e.g., coping with chronic illness or a learning disability) involved relationship challenges on a secondary level.

In both my professional and personal lives, I find that relationships are the greatest source of happiness and the greatest source of pain. On the positive side, when we are actively caring for and feel cared about by others, we simply feel and do better. Even in the face of external stressors beyond our control, the love, appreciation, and acceptance that come with healthy relationships decrease stress and build well-being.

So how can you make your relationships healthier? The most concrete way is with effective communication. Learning and practicing specific communication skills will help you interact more positively and effectively, decrease relationship stress, and help you feel more confident. Here are some specific communication skills, including assertiveness and conflict resolution, that I have found helpful in creating and repairing relationships.

SKILLS FOR STAYING CONNECTED

Communication skills include *thinking skills,* such as compassion voice and other strategies described earlier among the thought-change tools, and *actions,* for example, shaking a person's hand and saying something friendly to introduce yourself. In reality, the two skills interact so much that they are sometimes difficult to distinguish. (Remember how when Marisol thought compassionately about her difficult coworker at the hospital, her compassionate thoughts made it easier for her to act kindly toward her coworker, and the coworker's positive response increased Marisol's positive feeling toward her, which made it even easier to behave kindly.) Although we're now focusing specifically on action steps, as you will see, the thought-change tools interact with and augment the action, and vice versa.

VERBAL–BEHAVIORAL MATCH

The action part of communication includes both verbal and behavioral (i.e., nonverbal) elements. When a person is communicating effectively, their verbal and behavioral messages usually match (I say *usually* because humor often involves a deliberate mismatch). This verbal–behavioral match can be described as *genuineness* and is perceived as a sign of one's honesty and trustworthiness.

When a person says something that does not match what they're doing, we often feel confused, irritated, or distrustful—even if we know the person to be trustworthy. For example, I used to have an agency coworker who smiled constantly, even when she was talking about a difficult, sad, or negative topic. I knew her to be a kind and well-intentioned person, and it seemed that her smile was either out of nervousness or a defense against people who might not like her or something she'd done. But whenever I talked with her about a painful topic, I had to keep reminding myself to listen to the content of what she was saying, or I would be thrown off by her smile and then start to feel annoyed.

The behavioral messages we send via our behavior can weaken, contradict, or completely cancel our intended verbal message. For example, if you ask your partner the question "Do you want to go to that restaurant again?" the verbal part of the message communicates an interest in knowing his or her preference. However, the behavioral components of the message—your voice tone, volume, body language, gestures, eye contact, and even an emphasis on one word—may communicate something else.

> **Statement:** (with smiling, cheerful tone) "Do you want to go to that restaurant again?"
>
> **Underlying message:** *I am genuinely interested in your restaurant preference.*
>
> **Same statement:** (with rolling eyes, exasperated tone, emphasis on the word *again*) "Do you want to go to that restaurant again?"
>
> **Underlying message:** *I hate that restaurant, and if I have to go there one more time, you're going to owe me big.*

The point here is to pay attention to your own verbal—behavioral congruence, to be sure you're not undermining your intention with contradictory messages. In addition, if you're in an interaction and begin to feel defensive, annoyed, or distrustful, notice whether the other person's behavior is contradicting what he or she is saying; if it is, in some situations it may decrease the tension to simply restate the person's message and ask if you've got it right. When this feels awkward, another approach is to use one of the thought-change strategies to decrease your irritation. For example, with my smiling coworker, I reminded myself of what a kind and gentle person she was and told myself that she probably smiled without awareness because she wanted people to like her.

ACTIVE LISTENING

One of my favorite sayings from yoga class is: *We hear with our ears, but we listen with our hearts.* If you have even one person in your life who genuinely listens to you, you know what a gift it is. Although you can't control how well another person listens to you, you can communicate more effectively by giving the gift of actively listening to others. And in most cases, your efforts will be rewarded by a positive response.

Active listening involves paying close attention to what the person is saying—not thinking ahead about what you want to say. It requires focusing on the individual, including with your body language and behavior, and avoiding distraction from the surrounding environment. If this is difficult, it can help to mentally repeat the person's words to yourself as the person is speaking.

Active listening also involves some sort of response, whether it's a nod, a look, a question, or an uh-huh, or paraphrasing back what the person has just said. *Paraphrasing* consists of restating what the person has said either in the form of a question or with something like, "So I hear you saying . . . " or "It sounds like you're saying . . . "

There are family and cultural differences with active listening, and I will mention one in particular because it's the one I most commonly come across that can stop a relationship before it starts—verbal *interrupting*. The following is an example of well-intentioned interrupting.

> *Person A:* Do you know the name of that store that sells the flowers that have . . .
>
> *Person B:* You mean those flowers that are the really good fakes? It's over by that two-story building. It's the one with the . . .
>
> *Person A:* Oh, yeah, the building with the yellow awning where that guy always . . .
>
> *Person B:* Yeah, the guy who always wears that big yellow hat that matches the awning that . . .
>
> *Person A:* Yeah, yeah, that's it. Do you think he does that on purpose to match?

In some families and cultures, this kind of interrupting is completely normal and communicates engagement. However, in other families and cultures, it is considered disrespectful and rude. For example, in traditional Alaska Native cultures, there is an expectation that before responding, the listener will pause for a second after the speaker finishes; this brief pause communicates respect for what the person has said and shows that the listener is not simply thinking about what they want to say in response. When you put two people with these different communication styles together, the interrupter often assumes that the pauser is mentally slow or hard of hearing, and the pauser thinks the interrupter is the rudest person they've ever met.

Marisol's physical sensations of increased tension and mild anxiety cued her to pay attention to what was going on in her

---

Consider This

Which speech pattern is the norm in your family and culture—interruptive or pausing between speakers? _____

Does this norm vary depending on a person's status, age, gender, or role in the family (e.g., OK for parents to interrupt children but not vice versa)?

_____

---

interactions with Anya, the difficult hospital administrator. Marisol noticed that every time she was interrupted by Anya, her tension increased a little more. To keep from becoming defensive and disconnecting from Anya, Marisol took a deep breath and told herself that Anya was "just wired" and obviously trying to connect. Later, as their relationship improved, she talked to Anya in a kind way about their different styles, then in the moment of an interruption, asked Anya to please let her finish.

ASSERTIVENESS

Assertiveness is *not* the same as aggressiveness, but people often confuse the two. It can help to think of them as existing on the same continuum, with a lack of assertiveness at one end, assertiveness in the middle, and aggressiveness at the other end. Assertiveness is in the middle because it involves a balance between letting people know your wants and needs when it feels appropriate, but at the same time considering other people's wants and needs. In contrast, aggression involves neglecting others' needs, whereas unassertiveness means consistently neglecting your own needs. I say "consistently neglecting" because there are times when putting others' needs before your own is the generous and appropriate thing to do.

Ironically, a lack of assertiveness can contribute to aggressive behavior. This happens when an individual tries to be unrealistically considerate, kind, and nice, and in repeated attempts to always be nice, the individual pushes down his or her own desires to the point of neglecting his or her own needs. Over time, those wants and needs build, until the individual eventually explodes at someone who has just made a fairly small request or a comment that the individual perceives as "the last straw." The person then feels horrible about the outburst and tries even harder to be nice, pushing down his or her preferences and needs again, in a continuous cycle.

As Carol became more aware of her own part in the negative interactions with her husband and daughter, she recognized this pattern in herself. A specific example occurred every time she and her husband decided to watch a movie together. Although Sal would ask her what she wanted to see, Carol nearly always said, "Oh, I don't care," and then they would either rent or go see the movie he chose. They interacted similarly with many other decisions too, including big purchases, travel plans, and holiday family gatherings.

Over the years, as Carol put Sal's, their kids', and his mother's preferences and needs ahead of her own, the pressure from her own unmet wishes continued to build. Periodically, she would explode over some minor request, such as Sal asking if she would fix him a cup of coffee. Then she would feel guilty, berate herself with hateful self-talk, and try harder to be helpful and considerate, which she thought meant going along with whatever the other person wanted, repeating the whole buildup again.

But as Carol began to understand the necessity of self-care to her well-being, she also recognized the importance of being more assertive regarding her wants and needs. She slowly began sharing her preferences and politely declining requests that took more time and energy than she wanted to give. This was hard for her to do, and she used self-talk to help her make these changes, repeatedly reminding herself that taking care of herself would help her to be a better wife, mother, grandmother, and person. She told herself that the people who cared about her genuinely wanted to know her thoughts and feelings, and letting them know what she preferred would improve her relationships over the long haul. She also talked with her husband and daughter about what she was trying to do. Although they were mostly support-ive, there were times when their desires conflicted and Carol needed to step up her self-talk to follow through with her own self-care.

CONFLICT RESOLUTION

Conflict is a normal occurrence in close relationships, including healthy ones. Whenever you put two people together for any length of time, there will eventually be some sort of disagreement. What matters is how you resolve the conflict when it occurs.

The most common block to effective conflict resolution is *defensiveness*—the cognitive and emotional rigidity that comes when a person feels threatened. Defensiveness can arise out of fear, a desire to avoid pain, or attachment to a particular outcome or desire. When we feel defensive, we cease to understand the other person and retreat into self-protection.

But remember the earlier point about unwanted feelings being helpful at times? This is true of *defensive feelings*. Although defensive *behaviors* can get you into trouble, defensive *feelings* can be helpful. Whether the defensive feeling is coming from you or the other person, you can use it as a signal that something is off in the interaction so you better pay attention to what's going on. The more mindful you are of your feelings and what triggers them, the more able you will be to respond thoughtfully rather than emotionally.

If you don't pay attention and let the feeling lead you into defensive behavior, then the defensive behavior will increase the stress on the interaction. Whether it's an overtly aggressive defensive behavior (e.g., talking louder, a patronizing tone, irritability) or a more subtle withdrawal from the other person, defensive behavior works against a positive connection. This is true whether the defensiveness arises first in you or in the other person, because defensiveness in one person usually elicits the same from the other. Of course, there are times when it may be appropriate to react defensively, for example, when you're in real physical danger. But if you are lucky enough to live in a politically and economically stable country and community, the threat is usually more mental or social than physical.

Consider This

List your defensive behaviors. If you think you don't have any, ask your best friend, partner, or a family member what your defensive behaviors are. _____

_____

DECREASING DEFENSIVENESS

When you notice defensiveness in an interaction, whether it is coming from you or the other person, the following steps can help you slow your emotional reaction, giving you time to think and behave in the most helpful way.

1. *Pay attention to your body.* Notice the physical sensations in your body and any thoughts associated with them. Use the sensations as cues regarding your emotions and what is going on in the interaction.
2. *Take a deep breath and exhale slowly, focusing on your breath.* This creates a little distance between you and your defensive feeling.

3. *Ask yourself,* What am I reacting to here? Is this defensive feeling coming from me, and if so, why? Or am I picking up on the other person's feeling? Am I doing or saying something that is contributing to their defensiveness?

4. *Refrain from defensive behaviors.* Imagine you are in a tug-of-war; if you keep pulling, the other person will too. To stop the tug-of-war, only one person needs to let go or back off, and that person can be you.

5. *Acknowledge the other person's point* by paraphrasing and asking if you've understood correctly. Often a defensive interaction can be stopped if even one person shows they are trying to understand the other's perspective, because when a person feels understood and accepted, there is no need to defend (even if there is disagreement).

6. Re-*place the problem.* Instead of thinking of the person as the problem, imagine the problem sitting in the physical space in front of you and the person and looking for a solution together.

7. *Question your need for matching views.* Ask yourself, *What am I so attached to here or wanting to happen? What is more important—maintaining a good connection with this person or being right?*

8. *Recognize that you may need additional information or experiences.* If it applies, take the generous route and tell the other person that you need more information or experience to understand their perspective.

As Sheldon thought more about his part in the breakup with his girlfriend, he began to recognize how his reaction to her concerns about his work schedule worked against resolving their conflicts. In retrospect, he could see that when she asked about getting together with friends or going out, he frequently tensed up and told her in an irritable tone that he had too much to do. If she pressed, he would say something sharp, such as "I SAID I can't!" then withdraw from her. Although he considered his withdrawing to be helpful because it stopped them from arguing, in reality his defensive reaction pushed her away and allowed him to avoid the issue.

Although Sheldon couldn't change the past, he began to watch for this defensive response toward coworkers who wanted something from him. He realized that although an irritable comment got him what he wanted (i.e., the person backed off), in the long run it worked against him by pushing people away. So when he noticed the feeling of irritation in himself, he would take a deep breath and look up from whatever he was doing to give the person his full attention. Even if he could not give them what they wanted, this simple act of carefully listening and responding respectfully made him feel better and improved his work relationships.

In sum, although agreement is usually the goal of conflict resolution, agreement is not always possible. In such cases, keeping a positive connection is a good second best. A positive connection involves your best attempt at listening, understanding, and accepting the other person as he or she is.

FIVE MORE DO'S AND DON'TS FOR GOOD COMMUNICATION

Here are a few more miscellaneous tips on communication that will help you build better relationships.

Do's

1. *Reach out.* Most people wait for others to initiate conversation and get-togethers, which is probably why so many people experience loneliness in spite of all the people around them. Ask about the other person with genuine interest and remember what the person says. Then the next time you see the person, ask how it's going regarding that particular topic.

2. *Match the mood.* If the other person is feeling blue, sympathize first before you try more positive conversation. Once a person feels understood, he or she will often move on to another subject.

3. *Be positive.* You will make more friends if you make more positive comments than negative ones, discuss topics that are enjoyable for others, and avoid negative comments about others that can come back to bite you.

4. *Wear a whatzit.* A *whatzit* is an unusual tie, pin, hairpiece, jewelry, or article of clothing that invites comments from others (Lowndes, 2003). It gives others an easy way to start a conversation with you, for example, "That's an interesting pin. Where did you get that?" Have an interesting bit of information ready to tell about your whatzit. You can also use it to show you have a sense of humor, as people love to share a laugh.

5. *Give a little information,* enough that the other person has something to tack a comment onto. For example, when people used to ask my husband, "What do you do?" he would say, "I'm retired," which tended to stop the conversation. Since realizing this was happening, he now says, "I worked in several positions in education throughout Alaska," and people usually respond with "Oh, where in Alaska?" or "What kind of positions?" which starts the conversation rolling.

Don'ts

1. *Don't ask "What do you do?"* When you first meet someone, this question can feel to the other person like you're assessing his or her status relative to yours. Also, not everyone has a job they like to talk about or that others find interesting. An alternative is, "What do you like to do in your spare time?"

2. *Don't brag.* My sister uses the following saying to help her feel less annoyed at a coworker who brags incessantly: *He who sings his own praises is usually a soloist.*

3. *Don't joke at someone else's expense.* No laugh is worth hurting someone's feelings.

4. *Don't repeat yourself.* Say it once and then let the other person talk.

5. *Don't share too much about yourself right away.* When you share a lot of personal information in an initial meeting, you may be perceived as self-centered and needing to talk about yourself. Focus instead on getting to know the other person. Ask about the person's perspective, experiences, or interests.

SMALL STEP

Pick a communication skill that you would like to improve, and practice it for a week. Watch for how using this skill affects your feelings, thoughts, and relationships.

CHAPTER 14

SOCIAL ENGAGEMENT, MEANING, AND PURPOSE

We make a living by what we get. We make a life by what we give.

—Winston Churchill

We humans are social creatures, and relationships are essential to our survival and well-being. Social engagement that includes being cared for and caring for others is key to a life of meaning and purpose.

On the 99-square-mile Greek island of Ikaria, inhabitants reach the age of 90 at a rate of 2½ times that of the United States, have a quarter the rate of dementia, and experience less depression. Researchers have pinpointed a number of factors contributing to the Ikarians' health, such as their Mediterranean diet; moderate consumption of red wine; herbal teas with medicinal properties; physical activity related to farm work and living amid hills; and a natural rhythm to work and life that includes daily social activities, sleeping late, and regular naps. But most important is what seems to keep these health-producing activities in place: Tight-knit communities, in which members are actively engaged in caring for one another, reinforce the communal values and lifestyle. As one resident noted, "It's not a 'me' place. It's an 'us' place" (Buettner, 2012).

You can follow all the expert-recommended exercise, dietary, sleep, and other health practices to a "T," but without strong relationships, they won't make you happy. Social engagement that includes giving and receiving support brings meaning and purpose to our daily activities. Research has suggested that social structure—those mutually reinforcing relationships that build and support healthy choices and lifestyles—have a profound influence on well-being (Buettner, 2012).

In the previous chapter, we looked at assertiveness and other communication skills for building healthy relationships (the *A* in the CLASS action steps). Now let's look at some additional strategies for engaging in relationships more mindfully and appreciatively, in ways that increase the richness of your life and enhance the well-being of those around you.

SOCIAL SUPPORT, STRESS, AND HEALTH

People are often surprised when I say that going through a divorce was much harder for me than being diagnosed with breast cancer. I think what accounts for the differences were my two different social situations. During the divorce, I was living far from my family, my closest friends had recently moved, and I was in a city apartment where I didn't know my neighbors. In contrast, by the time I was diagnosed with cancer, I was back living in my small Alaskan hometown near family and my dearest high school friend, in a happy second marriage, and connected via phone and Internet to friends who regularly called and sent messages of support. In sum, I felt tremendously loved, and this feeling somehow lessened or countered the fear, anxiety, fatigue, and physical pain I endured.

My experience is one that has been backed up by numerous studies documenting the stress-reducing and pain-countering effects of support. In one such study, women undergoing a frightening medical procedure experienced less anxiety if someone simply held their hand. Brain scans showed a corresponding decrease in activity in the part of the brain that lights up in response to fear. If the hand-holder was the woman's husband and the marriage was a loving one, the anxiety-reducing effect was even greater than when the person was a stranger (Coan, Schaefer, & Davidson, 2005).

In another study of pain perception, participants were asked to bring in a photo of an acquaintance or a loved one and look at it during a procedure in which their palms were heated to an uncomfortable level. Looking at the acquaintance's photo had no effect on participants' pain level during the procedure; however, when the photo was of a loved one, participants reported a reduction in pain, and brain imaging showed increased activity in the brain's reward center (Younger, Aron, Parke, Chatterjee, & Mackey, 2010).

Not only is social support a buffer against stress and pain, it also seems to increase psychological and physical health. In a study conducted at the University of Rochester, researchers found that happily married husbands and wives who had heart bypass surgery were up to 3 times more likely than their unmarried counterparts to be alive 15 years later (Love Helps, 2011). Positive, supportive relationships reduce the risk of health problems ranging from the common cold to stroke to various psychological disorders, and they are correlated with greater happiness, resilience, cognitive capacity, and quality of life (Walsh, 2011).

SOCIAL ENGAGEMENT AND WELL-BEING

Whereas the health risks of social isolation are on par with those of obesity, smoking, and high blood pressure (Walsh, 2011), social *engagement* that includes receiving and *giving* support has been repeatedly linked to happiness, health, and well-being. As in the case of Ikaria, socially engaged people feel and *are* needed by others. They have a reason to get up in the morning, and they persist in the face of obstacles because they care. This sense that one is an integral, needed part of a larger whole is, at the same time, a source of support.

In their book about an 8-decades-long study of 1,500 people beginning in 1921, Howard S. Friedman and Lesley R. Martin (2011) found that contrary to popular ideas about a stress-free life of retiring early and relaxing on a Florida beach, those who stayed actively involved in meaningful work and *worked the hardest* lived the longest, healthiest lives. As the authors found, hard work and social challenges do not necessarily produce the chronic physiological disturbance we call stress; the individuals who thrive are those dedicated to things and people beyond themselves.

In addition to the positive effects of sharing and caring on health and longevity, giving behavior has immediate positive effects. In one study demonstrating this effect, participants were given $20, and half of them were told to buy themselves a treat while the other half were told to buy a gift for someone else. Afterward, both groups were asked to rate their happiness, and the group that spent the money on someone else reported greater happiness (Dunn, Aknin, & Norton, 2008). On a broader scale, studies conducted at the University of Stony Brook involving more than 1,900 adults found that people enjoyed spending their discretionary money more if they spent it on social activities (Caprariello & Reis, 2013).

WIRED FOR CONNECTION

Psychologists use the term *attunement* to describe people's strong connection to, and influence on, one another. Individuals who are highly attuned to one another often sense what the other is feeling, and the well-being of one affects the well-being of the other. In the study I cited earlier of women holding either a stranger's or their husband's hand during a scary medical procedure, one additional finding was that although the women could not see *who* was holding their hand, they always guessed correctly who it was (Coan, Schaefer, & Davidson, 2005). I call this attunement.

Neuroscientists have recently discovered the brain mechanism that facilitates attunement: *mirror neurons*. In a study illustrating how mirror neurons work, a laser-thin electrode was inserted into a single neuron of an awake person to monitor their neural response to a pinprick. Results showed that the neuron fired when the person anticipated the pinprick and when the person simply *observed* someone else receiving a pinprick (Goleman, 2006).

Mirror neurons explain why we feel sad when we see someone else grieving, or we feel compelled to smile when a stranger smiles at us. The brain literally mimics what we observe others doing and saying, which in turn influences how we feel. Mirror neurons enable us to experience empathy and compassion, which are crucial to positive social engagement.

MINDFUL SOCIAL ENGAGEMENT

One way to enrich your life is by bringing mindfulness to your relationships. Such mindfulness involves thinking *deliberately* and *generously* about your relationships. Thinking *deliberately* means paying attention to the daily interactions you have, including interactions with people you may not think about—for example, the cashier at the grocery store, the bank teller, the barista who fixes your coffee, the bus driver, the dry cleaning attendant, the waitress at your lunch table, and so on.

My husband, Bob, is one of the best people I know at this. When I come into the room and he's talking on the phone, I can't tell whether he's talking to one of his closest friends or someone he's never met because he's always chatting with them in the same friendly tone, using their name and asking how their day has been going. One time when I called an Alaskan airline to make reservations for the two of us and I told the ticket agent his name, she said, "Oh, yeah, Bob, we know him!" Bob remembers the names of hotel desk clerks in places we visit once a year and generously gives compliments to people on their "excellent help." I think his genuine interest in every person he meets comes from years of living in remote Alaskan communities where every single individual is important.

The other part of mindful social engagement, thinking *generously* about relationships, involves recognizing the support you already have. For example, meditation teacher Thich Nhat Hanh once described his deep appreciation for all of the support he experienced while traveling. He was grateful for friendly, fellow passengers; a helpful ticket agent; responsible, hardworking flight attendants; and conscientious pilots who safely landed the plane—support that most people consider minor or take for granted. I imagine that whenever he travels, this appreciative attitude evokes a warm feeling from those around him, increasing the positive effect.

Try This: Mindful Connection

Think about a person you have regular contact with but know little or nothing about and imagine what their life is like. Ask yourself these kinds of questions:

Do they have a best friend?
Do or did their parents love them?
How do they feel about their work?
Do they have hopes and dreams for the future?
What is their deepest pain?

The next time you see this person, ask, "How is your day going?" (not "How are you?" which usually gets an autoresponse). Listen to the person's answer and respond, then think about these questions again.

To think more deliberately and generously about your social support, imagine your social relationships like an onion. The inner core of the onion includes your closest confidants with whom you can share anything, who are always there for you when you need them, and who love you for who you are. The next layer includes individuals who love and support you but not quite as reliably or regularly as the inner core. The next layer includes those who provide occasional support but not as reliably. Think of all these people as the layers of an onion. If you need to make the onion bigger, you can add as many layers as you need.

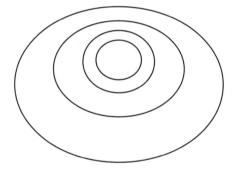

The point of the exercise above is to become more appreciative of a wide range of relationships in your life, and the different things you receive from them. If you tend toward black-and-white thinking when it comes to relationships (e.g., *A true friend is either there for me or they're not*), this exercise can help you change your approach. Instead of cutting someone out of your life because they are not 100% reliable, appreciate what you *do* receive from them, and then consider adding new people and layers to your onion by developing new relationships. To further increase your mindfulness of the support you receive, try the exercise below.

Thinking more specifically about the kind of support you receive from important individuals in your life may increase your attitude of gratitude, or it may call to your attention some areas in which you need extra help. It might also explain why you feel frustrated with a lack of support, for example, if it's clear that you are relying on one person for all of your support.

Try This: Receiving Support

Fill in the names of the five people you consider your closest friends or family members—the innermost layers of your onion. (If you have more, feel free to make a longer list.) Now put a check mark under the kind of support each person gives you. The *physical* category refers to practical needs, such as helping you move, giving you a ride, or taking care of you when you are sick.

	Name	Financial	Physical	Emotional	Advice	Fun	Other
Person 1							
Person 2							
Person 3							
Person 4							
Person 5							

When Marisol did these exercises and began thinking about her relationships more mindfully, she felt a little better. She realized how many people she could count on for support, even if she rarely did so. Recognizing that these people would help her if she asked them—to varying degrees depending on who they were—decreased her anxiety a little. She also noticed that when her stress level was higher, as it had been the past few months, she depended more on her partner, Kate, and less on friends for emotional support, advice, and fun. She realized that, at times, this was expecting too much of Kate, and it would help their relationship to vent more with her friends and get advice from them too.

In an effort to be more mindful, Marisol also decided to make a deliberate effort to interact with the front desk receptionist at the hospital where she worked, who she had not thought about before, possibly because the position had such high turnover. She was pleasantly surprised by the receptionist's warm response, which gave her a little mood boost as she was entering the building to start her day.

Of course, social *engagement* is a two-way street, so below is one more exercise to help you look at the other side of social support—what you're giving back. If you have five mutually supportive relationships that provide you with plenty of support, that's great. But in addition to these mutual relationships, there may also be some people with whom the support is one way, from you to them. Sharing time and resources with people who are unable to share back is part of being socially engaged, and studies show that this kind of social engagement builds well-being in the giver. People who engage in and enjoy volunteering over the course of their lives live longer and healthier lives.

Try This: Giving Support

Return to your Receiving Support checklist and put a plus sign under the kind of support you *give* each of these people. Those who have both checks and plus signs next to their names are your *mutually supportive* relationships.

One-way support is usually the expectation for people who work or volunteer in health care, education, social services, and other helping professions or who donate to helping organizations. If the work is too demanding, the result may be compassion fatigue and caregiver burnout. However, if the situational demands match the ability to give, such work has big rewards. My 80-year-old mom, who volunteers for three different organizations, says that one of the reasons she does so is that since retiring from her position as a college professor, she no longer has as many opportunities for helping others, and she learned long ago that giving, sharing, and helping are the greatest sources of joy and happiness.

Although Sheldon's agreement to coach the kids' basketball team was only partly motivated out of a desire to help others, he still reaped the benefits. The kids made him laugh, and he had fun with them. He started looking forward to the three evenings of practice per week and to the weekend games, which in turn displaced some of his obsessive thinking and compulsive behavior regarding work. And the appreciation he received from the parents and a couple of teachers increased his desire to be even more helpful.

Unlike Sheldon, who hadn't previously thought about volunteering, Carol had long lived a life of service. She received many benefits from caring for others, including love, appreciation, and support. However, she went just a little too far on the helping continuum, past her own physical and psychological limits. She liked thinking of this issue as a matter of balance, between enacting her values of being a helper and contributor while at the same time validating her need for self-care. The better she became at balancing these two approaches, the more enjoyable her helping behavior felt.

ENGAGING WITH DIFFICULT PEOPLE

During my years of working as a cross-cultural psychologist, I have come to believe that the most important common denominator for positive social engagement is *respect*. Although two people may disagree on an issue, including the morality or immorality of a particular belief or behavior, if both people treat one another with respect, a positive connection can be formed.

One advantage to treating someone respectfully is that you usually get the respect back (and if you treat someone disrespectfully, it's almost certain you'll get disrespect back). In addition, acting respectfully positively affects how you feel about yourself. I like the American Indian approach to respect: Unlike the dominant culture, which expects people to earn respect, traditional Native people give respect to everyone and everything because being respectful is the best way of being and of living in harmony with the world.

Respect opens the door to compassion, another powerful social facilitator. But with some especially difficult people, compassion may be more difficult, and respect is all you can give. Here are some suggestions for developing and sustaining respectful relationships, even with difficult people. You may notice that many of these also build compassion.

1. *Common interest.* Look for an interest, value, or relationship you have in common with the other person. Focus (in your mind and in your comments) on this shared experience or viewpoint in your daily interactions with the person.

2. *Different shoes.* Imagine being the other person, and as you do so, try thinking about their annoying behavior or your conflict with them from their perspective. Use the *most generous interpretation technique* (from Chapter 8) when you're imagining their perspective. Imagine, without defending your own position, how and why they see *you* as the difficult one.

3. *Acts of kindness.* Sometimes the simplest act of kindness can overcome hurt feelings. Even if the other person responds unkindly, remember the example of kindness in the values exercise: *What would a kind person do in this situation?*

Remind yourself that if you respond with hostility, you are letting the other person shape your behavior into that of someone you don't want to be.

4. *My favorite aunt.* Pretend that the annoying person is your favorite, much older aunt (or similar beloved elder). Talk to the person in the same caring and respectful way you would talk with your aunt. Remind yourself that just as you and your aunt have had vastly different experiences that have shaped what you believe and what you do, so have you and this other person.

5. *Everyone's my teacher.* Think of the difficult person as teaching you something about yourself. This is a variation of the growth opportunity tool described earlier, in which you ask yourself, *What can I learn about myself from my reactions to this person?*

SMALL STEP

Think of a person who bugs the heck out of you, and practice one of these tools with them. If you don't notice any change in your feeling toward the person with one tool, try another tool. Remember that anything you do to repair a difficult relationship benefits you too.

Alternatively, volunteer your time or resources to help someone else and watch for how your volunteering affects how you feel in the moment and any other positive effects on your thoughts, feelings, behavior, or relationships.

CHAPTER 15

SELF-CARE FOR STAYING ON THE HAPPY, HEALTHY PATH

The seeds that are watered grow.

—Thich Nhat Hanh

Good self-care is key to maintaining positive change. Some self-care activities require willpower, and some are so enjoyable that they are easy to do. Well-being requires both.

Bernice Bates is a mentally and physically healthy woman who, at 5 feet 2 inches and 104 pounds, attributes her flexibility, fitness, and all-around health to yoga (Flam, 2011). When Bernice began doing yoga, I doubt that her long-term goal was to do it for 60 years. But one day added to the next until here she is, at 91, still practicing and teaching yoga.

Health and longevity do not depend so much on the huge decisions we obsess over, but rather on the daily little decisions and actions that shape who we become. This means that, as in the case of Bernice, every little step you take in the direction of well-being adds to your previous steps, which over time build your happiness and health. So far, we've looked at steps toward *thinking* more positively and realistically with the thought-change tools, and the CLASS *action* steps to Create a healthier environment, Learn and practice behaviors that build well-being, use communication skills such as Assertiveness to improve relationships, and engage Socially to increase the richness of your life and share your well-being with others. Now in this last chapter, we'll look at the final action step: Self-care.

ENGAGING IN SELF-CARE

Good self-care involves more than showering and brushing your teeth; it includes caring for yourself the way you would care for a child, with consideration for your mind, body, and spirit. In my clinical practice, I have found that self-care is especially difficult for caregivers who have put the needs of partners, children, and/ or adult parents first for so long that they consider taking care of themselves selfish. But in reality, people who take care of themselves have more energy to help others. As the flight attendant advises, you need to put your own oxygen mask on before you help other people with theirs. The more consistently you take care of yourself, the easier it is to maintain a healthy balance between caring for yourself and helping others.

I divide self-care into two categories: the ones that are easy because they are enjoyable and the challenging ones that take effort and willpower. Following the path of least resistance, let's start with the easiest.

EASY SELF-CARE

There are many small self-care activities that cost little or no money and involve minimal effort and no new learning. With these types of self-care, all that is needed is to give yourself permission to do them.

You can use the list you create in the exercise on p. 182 in three ways. First, when you feel stressed, you can simply do these activities, working your way down the list until your stress decreases. Or you can consider adding at least one of these activities to your daily

Try This

Circle the activities that feel nurturing to you. Easy self-care activities are person specific. These are just a few examples to get you thinking about what works as self-care for *you.*

a walk outside

burning a scented candle

a warm blanket in your favorite
chair

herbal tea in your favorite cup

reading the funnies

snuggling with your partner

petting your dog or cat

painting your nails

laughing and playing with kids

watching a funny movie

reading a good book

buying your favorite magazine

a special dinner

fresh-cut flowers

a favorite food

morning devotions, prayer

meditation

sitting outdoors

fleece clothing

listening to your favorite
music

listening to an inspirational talk

going out to eat

creating, growing, or building
something

talking with/calling a friend

planning a fun trip

planning something to look forward
to

gardening

fishing

a support group

counseling

massage

a religious meeting/group

watching/feeding birds

painting, drawing

routine to increase your general well-being. Last, you can use individual activities as rewards to reinforce desired behavior change.

For some people, particular self-care activities lead to an experience known as *flow* (Csikzentmihalyi, 2008). Also known as *being in the zone*, flow has been described as the rapturous joy experienced when one is completely focused on and in alignment with a particular activity, such as sailing, playing music,

---

Try This

On the lines below (or on your electronic device), make your own easy self-care list, including the activities you circled in the previous exercise and any additional ones, keeping in mind your physical, mental, emotional, and spiritual needs. List your activities in order of what's the *most* nurturing thing for you as #1, the second most nurturing as #2, and so on.

My Easy Self-Care Activities

1. _____	11. _____
2. _____	12. _____
3. _____	13. _____
4. _____	14. _____
5. _____	15. _____
6. _____	16. _____
7. _____	17. _____
8. _____	18. _____
9. _____	19. _____
10. _____	20. _____

---

gardening, and artwork *or* as a complete absence of emotions while engaged in the activity. Either way, it is an experience that people treasure. Flow is characterized by

- immersion in the activity that is so focused you lose your sense of self and awareness of bodily needs (e.g., of being hungry or thirsty while engaged);
- time distortion, for example, when engaged in the activity, 5 hours go by but feel like 15 minutes;
- a desire to engage in the activity that is so strong you'll make sacrifices to engage in it, for example, the woman who loves

to ski so much that she works at a restaurant job she doesn't like because it allows her to live at the ski resort;

- clear goals that give the activity direction and structure; and
- a continuous learning process in which you're always challenged to learn or do a little more.

Sheldon made playing basketball his first step toward well-being because he had experienced flow in the past when he was on a team. He knew that when he played basketball regularly, time flew by; he didn't notice feeling hungry; and the more he played, the better he got. His decision is a good example of how one small self-care step, even if it is a fun one, can easily lead into others. Playing 1 night each week improved Sheldon's mood a little, gave him some exercise, and created the opportunity to coach the kids' team. In turn, coaching the kids' team 3 nights a week decreased his drinking and obsessive thinking about work, which further improved his mood, which improved his interactions with coworkers.

If you experience flow while engaged in an activity that you enjoy, this is probably the self-care activity for you. But whether you experience flow or not, it is important to have fun and leisure time in your life. Although fun activities are often the first to be dropped when we feel overwhelmed with work and other pressures, during stressful situations, they are especially important because they counter the experience of stress.

Consider learning to do one of these activities listed in the box above. It is OK to learn and do the activity in a way that involves minimal effort; that is, you do not have to invest the time and energy that are usually involved to experience flow, unless you are ready for a really big step. The main point is to have fun and enjoy yourself.

> **Try This: Fun Activities That Can Bring Flow**
>
> Circle any activity that sounds interesting or enjoyable to you now, and add any others that you can think of.
>
> | | | |
> |---|---|---|
> | sailing | math puzzles | playing music |
> | skiing | crosswords | gardening |
> | snowshoeing | writing | fishing |
> | walking | painting | scuba |
> | hiking | drawing | yoga |
> | climbing | pottery | origami |
> | surfing | crafts | photography |
> | cooking | beading | building |
> | sewing | dancing | learning a language |
> | quilting | singing | learning to fly a plane |
> | others: | | |

CHALLENGING SELF-CARE: THE BIG THREE

Not all self-care activities are fun or easy. The ones I call the *Big Three* require a lot of effort, but their payoff is enormous because even a small step can create a snowball of positive effects. The Big Three are *sleep, diet,* and *exercise*—all of which require self-control and discipline. So before getting into suggestions for improving each, you might want to know these recent findings on willpower.

First, the bad news: Recent research has shown that willpower is a limited resource. A study conducted by psychologist Roy Baumeister and his colleagues showed how the depletion of willpower works (Muraven, Baumeister, & Tice, 1999). A group of students was invited to eat chocolate chip cookies while a second group was asked to resist the cookies and snack on radishes instead. Both groups were then asked to solve a difficult geometry puzzle. Although the cookie eaters persisted on their puzzle for about 20 minutes, the group that resisted the cookies gave up on the puzzle after only 8 minutes. Apparently resisting the cookies decreased the second group's ability to persist with the difficult puzzle.

More bad news: On average, each of us spends 3 or 4 hours per day resisting desires, with additional time spent making decisions, regulating task performance, and controlling emotions. All of these behaviors involve an element of self-control. During an especially stressful morning, we may spend all of our willpower even before the free afternoon donuts arrive in the lunchroom.

Now for the good news: It *is* possible to increase willpower! One of the simplest ways is via glucose. During digestion, our body breaks down the carbohydrates we eat into glucose, which acts as fuel for the body and brings energy to the brain, increasing the ability to exert self-control. Of course, this is a problem if what you are trying to resist is food.

For a more lasting effect, self-control can be strengthened with exercise. As with occasional *physical* exercise that leaves you feeling exhausted, the occasional use of *self-control* results in an immediate depletion of willpower. However, just as regular physical exercise gradually builds muscle and strength, practicing self-control regularly increases willpower in as little as 2 weeks (Weir, 2012).

Self-control exercises may be specific to the behavior you want to change; for example, practicing resistance to impulse buying will increase your willpower to resist impulse buying. But amazingly, research has shown that self-control practice is also helpful when it is *unrelated* to the desired behavior change. For example, regularly practicing good posture, or using your nondominant hand to brush your teeth, will improve your self-control for other desired changes. This probably explains why people who are disciplined in one area of their life often have good self-control in other areas too.

Try This: Building Willpower

1. Think of a behavior you want to change. Make it a measurable behavior, for example, eating fewer desserts, smoking fewer cigarettes, exercising 5 minutes longer per day, studying an extra 10 minutes per day, watching 30 minutes of television per day, or buying a less expensive coffee drink once per day.

   _____

2. Rate your willpower regarding this behavior on a scale of 0 (*no self-control over this behavior*) to 10 (*total control*):_____.
3. Name a self-control exercise you could engage in for 2 weeks—either the behavior you are wanting to change or an unrelated behavior:_____. Practice the exercise daily and at the end of 2 weeks, rate your self-control for the specific behavior again: _____.

Let's turn now to The Big Three self-care activities. As you think about the changes you want to make with regard to sleep, diet, or exercise, remember the *Seven Behavior Change Rules* including the SMART approach (i.e., goals that are Specific, Measurable, Achievable, Relevant, and Time-framed; see Chapter 12).

Sleep

Around the time I turned 40, I lost my previous ability to sleep 10 hours straight and started waking up for 2 hours in the middle of the night even when I wasn't worried about anything. I tried everything I could to counter this (except medication, because I know sleep medication can be addictive), but nothing worked. Then I came across the following study by the National Institute of Mental Health, which completely changed my feelings about my 2-hour insomnia episodes (Wylie, 2008).

In the study, participants lived for several weeks in winter-simulated conditions of 14 hours of darkness per 24-hour cycle. Over time, the participants developed a common sleep pattern of about 2 hours of wakeful rest (i.e., lying in bed with eyes closed) followed by 4 to 5 hours of sleep, then 2 or 3 more hours of wakeful rest and 4 or 5 hours of sleep. Researchers concluded that we human beings need *rest* as much as we need sleep. However, because we live in a world of artificial light that is manipulated according to work and other demands, we compress our sleep/rest needs into a sleep-only schedule. The average adult sleeps about 6.5 hours per night, and doesn't even think about rest. We go full steam and then, if we're lucky, fall asleep and stay asleep (because we're sleep deprived) until the alarm clock goes off.

When we are young, our bodies adapt more easily to artificially imposed sleep/wake schedules. But as we age, our bodies are less able to adapt, and we have more trouble falling asleep and staying asleep. Expecting to go-go-go right up to bedtime and then boom—fall asleep—is like driving your car 80 mph into the garage and expecting to be able to come to a full stop (Wylie, 2008). Inadequate sleep over time is extremely stressful to the mind and body and contributes to anxiety, depression, irritability, hypertension, heart disease, obesity, impaired reasoning, lowered immune system function, and heightened awareness of pain.

So now when I have my 2-hour wake-up, I tell myself that I must be getting enough sleep, but I still need to rest. Sometimes while I'm lying there I meditate, and sometimes I write part of a book chapter in my head, but I don't get stressed out about it anymore.

When you consider all of the media stimulation, energy drinks, 24-hour availability of consumer goods, and the technological bells and whistles bombarding us minute by minute, it's no wonder we have trouble falling and staying asleep. Following are a few suggestions of natural ways to aid sleeping *and* resting:

1. *Avoid caffeinated beverages several hours before bedtime.* These include energy drinks.
2. *Exercise every day,* because exercise releases the physical tension that develops in response to stress. (However, avoid exercising right before bedtime.)
3. *Keep regular hours.* In studying the habit of staying up late and sleeping late on weekends, researcher Till Roenneberg used the term *social jet lag* to describe the physiological stress that people experience when their internal body clock is out of sync with the social clock set by morning alarms, bright lights, and the demands of work life. In a survey of 65,000 people, he and his colleagues found 69% to be suffering from at least 1 hour of social jet lag each week (Roenneberg, Allebrandt, Merrow, & Vetter, 2012).
4. Schedule 1 hour of "relax time" right before bed. Do something relaxing; for example, take a hot bath; meditate; listen to calming music; or read a magazine, newspaper, or book that you *can* put down. TV and computers are not a good idea because the bright light is energizing.
5. Save the bed for sleep and sex. If you work in bed, the bed becomes a cue for getting into work mode, and you don't want to be thinking about work when you're trying to fall asleep.
6. During the day, take rest breaks. Find a way to take 5 or 10 minutes to be still and allow your mind and body to relax, even if you are just sitting in a chair at your desk with your eyes closed.

Diet

A recent article on lifestyle and mental health published by the American Psychological Association summarized research linking diet to better academic performance in children, improved mental health, and a reduction in age-related cognitive decline (Walsh, 2011). The recommended diet

- consists predominately of multicolored fruits and vegetables;
- contains some fish, preferably cold deep-seawater fish such as salmon (excluding shark, swordfish, king mackerel, and tilefish, which have high mercury contents); and
- reduces excessive calories to avoid obesity.

Complementing this advice is a 2013 study published in *The New England Journal of Medicine* showing that diet can have an effect as powerful as medication on physical health, specifically in preventing heart attacks, strokes, and deaths from cardiovascular disease (Estruch, 2013). Similar to the recommendations in the previous list, the diet that showed the best results was a Mediterranean diet high in fruits, vegetables, and fish; supplemented with olive oil or nuts; and low in red meat, dairy, and processed foods. Interestingly, in this study the researchers did not set any calorie limit on the experimental or control groups, yet the diet was so successful in preventing cardiovascular problems that the study was terminated early.

If you are trying to change your eating habits, it can help to start by looking for *facilitators* (Behavior Change Rule #4). Specifically, studies show that environmental factors have a big influence on eating behaviors. For example, in one study, two groups were given bowls of tomato soup to eat, but the bowls of the second group were attached to a tube underneath the table that subtly refilled the bowl without participants' awareness (Wansink, Painter, & North, 2005). After 20 minutes, participants in both groups were asked to stop and rate how full they felt. The continuously refilled group ate 73% more than those with normal bowls but did not report feeling any fuller. Similarly, drinking from a wider glass and eating from a bigger plate led people to consume up to 30% more calories (Winerman, 2011).

In a different study, the appearance and location of food made a difference. Toward the goal of changing schoolchildren's food preferences, when researchers took fruit that had been dumped in an ugly metal bin near a steam table and arranged it artistically in a fruit basket with nice lighting, the fruit sales more than doubled. In another school, salad sales increased by 200% when researchers moved the salad bar next to the cash register (Winerman, 2011).

Harvard nutritionist Lillian Cheung and Thich Nhat Hanh (Nhat Hanh & Cheung, 2010) have offered a number of tips for mindful eating, some of which build on these ideas:

- unplug all electronic devices and focus on the food (don't eat on the run, in the car, or when doing something that distracts you from eating);
- create a calm, pleasing environment, for example, with a nicely set table, candles, or flowers;
- chew each bite thoroughly before taking another one;
- eat one meal per week in silence (this works better for adults than children); and
- try planting and growing something that you can eat, to increase your appreciation of the food.

Eating mindfully fit well with Marisol's goal of improving her health and bringing peace into her life. In addition to the changes she made to her own environment (e.g., the healthy snack drawer at work, not buying unhealthy snacks for home), she and Kate agreed that there would be no more TV or electronic devices at the dinner table—breakfast and lunch were exceptions, as a compromise with Marisol's daughters, who were not happy with the new rule. Although the teens' frustration initially made dinners unenjoyable, after several days of sticking with it, their resistance decreased, and all agreed they were sharing more about their daily experiences with one another.

If you are hoping to lose weight by changing your eating behavior, keep in mind that although research shows that most diets *do* lead to short-term weight loss, this weight loss is rarely maintained. When weight loss *is* maintained, research has suggested that exercise is key (Mann et al., 2007).

Exercise

The research on exercise and well-being is clear. Exercise has many positive physical effects, including increased strength, improved sleep, and the breakdown of *muscular armor* (chronic muscle tension that develops in response to stress). Exercise improves mood and decreases anxiety, depression, substance abuse, and eating disorders. It increases blood flow to the brain, reducing age-related cognitive decline. And the more you exercise, the stronger the positive effects on both mood and cognitive functioning (Walsh, 2011).

Illustrating these effects, one study assigned sedentary, depressed adults to four different groups: (a) supervised exercise, (b) home-based exercise, (c) an antidepressant medication, or (d) a placebo. After 4 months, the first three groups all had lower rates of depression than the placebo group (what you would expect). But at the 1-year follow-up, participants who had continued to exercise regularly had lower depression scores than those who did not exercise regularly (Blumenthal et al., 2007; Weir, 2011). Similar effects have been found in studies of anxiety (Smits & Otto, 2011). What is even more remarkable about exercise is its power to reduce *future stress*. Professor of kinesiology and health educator John Bartholomew, along with his colleagues, found that a 20-minute hard run or 45-minute walk provides a stress inoculation effect that lasts up to 2 hours.[1]

---

[1]John Bartholomew interviewed and cited in Jayson (2012).

If your primary goal with exercise is to lose weight, keep the following in mind: To stick with an exercise plan, it is better to focus on the *immediate* benefits of the exercise than on your long-range goal. For example, rather than focusing on losing 20 pounds, it is better to anticipate and look for the boost to your mood, reduction in physical pain with increasing blood flow to the muscles, or the physical feeling of relaxation that come immediately after exercising. If you focus primarily on the 20 pounds, you are apt to feel discouraged and give up because it takes so much longer to reach this goal.

When Carol decided to take 1 hour each day for self-care, she started with activities that were enjoyable. This decision was a good one (following the path of least resistance) because with her lifetime of caregiving, just thinking about self-care was hard enough. However, over time, Carol's need to improve her health increased (or rather, her *awareness* of the need to improve it), and she decided to start by walking outdoors for 30 minutes, three times each week. She asked Sal to join her, and after a couple of weeks, he agreed. Gradually their walking evolved into a nightly 1-hour walk after dinner. During cold weather, they went to a nearby gym and walked the track. Walking *together* was a good exercise facilitator because when one didn't feel like going, the other would talk him or her into it. Walking also had a snowball effect in that both Carol and Sal became more conscious of their health and together made some positive changes to their diet, and their shared activities and goals added positive feelings to their relationship.

When it comes to making these especially challenging behavior changes, remember that failure is not the opposite of success, but rather a part of the process. Failure can be helpful because it teaches you what *not* to do next time. If you fall off your well-being path, all you need to do is take a small step in the right direction to restart your snowball of positive change.

SMALL STEP

Pick a small self-care step that you are 100% sure you can do every day for 1 week. It can be an easy activity or one related to the Big Three. During the week, watch for positive results that you didn't expect—the snowball effect.

AFTERWORD

Success is the sum of small efforts, repeated day in and day out.
—Robert Collier

After 3 months of small steps, Marisol was happy with what she had accomplished. She still wanted to lose weight, but she kept her focus on building her health and sense of peace with the previously mentioned activities and by allowing herself to weigh only once a month. She also made a new rule for herself that she would not eat standing up, which kept her from eating mindlessly. She did not count calories but found she was losing about 2 pounds per month. Although she was not yet at her ideal weight, she used the thought-change tools to be more accepting of herself. Specifically, she countered her thoughts of *something's wrong with me* and *it's useless (to try)*, and she replaced them with encouraging thoughts about the importance of patience and reminders that her positive changes would build on themselves like interest compounding in a bank.

Toward her goal of bringing more peace into her life, she continued her monthly walk in the woods and, combined with her goal of getting healthier, began walking on her lunch hour with a friend 2 or 3 days each week. Reconnecting with her friends took some of the stress off of her relationship with her partner, Kate, and her daughters. As Marisol's interactions with her family became more positive, her anxiety decreased, and she stopped procrastinating about the task of addressing the girls' college needs. She talked with them realistically about how much she and Kate could help them financially, how much their father would add to the pot, and their need to start saving from their part-time jobs. As her stress level decreased, she also had more patience at work, including with Anya, the hospital administrator.

When she compared her current sense of well-being with where she had been 3 months ago, she could see her progress. She still hoped to start sketching and playing the piano again but recognized these activities would add too much to her current schedule; for now, she was happy with where she was along her path of well-being. To keep herself on track, Marisol kept her *Creating Well-Being* book by her bedside, and when she was feeling low, she would pick it up to remind herself of her strengths (by looking at her Personal Strengths Inventory), compassion voice, and the importance of self-care. Although she didn't purposefully think about enlisting Kate and friends to help her by reading the book too, they did, and her conversations with them further reinforced her commitment and reminded her of the power of social support. She, Kate, and their friends decided they would try to be like the people on the Greek island of Ikaria, supporting and reinforcing a healthy lifestyle for one another.

The positive effects of Sheldon playing basketball once a week grew exponentially once he agreed to coach the kids' team. Over time, his friendship with Joe grew, he became friends with some of the kids' parents, and he went out on several dates with women they introduced him to. He stopped drinking at home, and as his anger subsided, he stopped blaming his former girlfriend and thought more compassionately about her and about his own role in their breakup. He continued to take his work seriously but increasingly recognized and reminded himself that he didn't have to—and realistically couldn't—"do it all." As he felt better, including feeling less tension in his neck and shoulders, he became more aware of times when the tension would return and used it as a cue to take a deep breath, stop, and rethink whatever he was doing or saying. He kept his *Creating Well-Being* book at work, and when he was feeling really pressured, he would glance at it and the bright orange sticky note he'd used to mark the section on *shoulds* to remind himself that usually it was only *him* telling himself that he should or had to do something.

Sheldon recognized the areas in which he still needed to improve, namely, eating healthier, going to bed earlier, and worrying less about his job. He also still wanted to get married and have kids. But as he felt happier and had more to look forward to in each day, he focused less on what he didn't have and more on appreciating the good things, friends, and family currently in his life.

Carol was very satisfied with the changes she'd made, including her daily self-care activities, increased assertiveness, physical exercise, and improved diet. Although her husband Sal still wanted her home more, as she became happier, he became more positive and less critical of her work, which made her want to spend more time with him. After being home alone all day, Sal liked hearing about her workday, and she was especially appreciative when he began cooking healthy meals several nights each week.

Carol's increased assertiveness with her daughter initially created more friction between them, but over time her daughter's attitude shifted from one of expecting Carol to babysit to appreciating when she did agree to babysit. Carol still struggled with what she called her "knee-jerk caretaking reaction," but she told herself that even if she continued to have this tendency, given her childhood experiences, that didn't mean she had to act on the urge when it arose. She still did kind things for people, but because she was more conscious of her actions and the limits of her resources, she no longer felt resentful afterward.

To stay focused on her goals, Carol started a journal in which she wrote several times each week, often during her 1 hour of self-care time. She included her ongoing Thought Record and Personal Strengths Inventory in the journal, adding a strength or support whenever she noticed another one or someone pointed one out to her. She kept her *Creating Well-Being* book with the journal for times when she needed a refresher, particularly on self-compassion and the well-being boosters. She looked forward to growing better at balancing her own self-care with her caring for others and to learning and growing more intellectually and spiritually. At the same time, she began thinking about reducing her hours at work because she and Sal were getting along so much better.

As for me, I continue to use these tools and share them with friends and family. As I mentioned earlier, Bob and I have been doing our attitude of gratitude exercise for several years, and my family now uses it as a blessing when we get together for a meal. I regularly use compassion voice to help me stay connected to people I don't click with but with whom I want to keep a positive relationship. I try to reframe minor health problems as my body's wise messages telling me that I need to slow down and pay attention, and then in response I do some yoga, meditate, or go to bed early. When I'm awake for 2 hours in the middle of the night, I counter my fears about losing beloved family members with: *OK, is it really helping me to think about this?* When I'm sick and don't do so well with countering the negative thoughts, I try to use self-compassion, reminding myself of what I would tell someone I love. When it comes to work-related decisions (e.g., whether to commit to this project, speaking engagement, or take on more clients), I go back to my value priorities and think about what is most important to me and how I want to live. I'm not saying I do all of this perfectly, of course—but in my attempts to build well-being in myself and others, these tools have helped me enormously.

So in conclusion, thank you for taking the time to read and consider these tools I've shared with you. If any of this has helped or touched you or someone you know, I would be delighted to hear about it. I would also like to hear of any tools I've not mentioned that you have found helpful. I can be reached through my website at http://www.drpamelahays.com.

I wish you a happy, healthy life!

REFERENCES

Adams, C. E., & Leary, M. R. (2007). Promoting self-compassionate attitudes toward eating among restrictive and guilty eaters. *Journal of Social and Clinical Psychology, 26,* 1120–1144. doi:10.1521/jscp. 2007.26.10.1120

Azar, B. (2011, March). Oxytocin's other side: Oxytocin has garnered media attention for its potential as a social lubricant and as a treatment for autism and other disorders. But researchers warn it's no panacea. *Monitor on Psychology, 42*(3), 40–42. doi:10.1037/e517762011-018

Barasch, M. I. (2009). *The compassionate life: Walking the path of kindness.* San Francisco, CA: Berrett-Koehler.

Beck, A. T., Rush, A. J., Shaw, B. F., & Emery, G. (1979). *Cognitive therapy of depression.* New York, NY: Guilford Press.

Beck, A. T., Wright, F. D., Newman, C. F., & Liese, B. S. (1993). *Cognitive therapy of substance abuse.* New York, NY: Guilford Press.

Blumenthal, J. A., Babyak, M. A., Doraiswamy, P. M., Watkins, L., Hoffman, B. M., Barbour, K. A., . . . Sherwood, A. (2007). Exercise and pharmacotherapy in the treatment of major depressive disorder. *Psychosomatic Medicine, 69,* 587–596. doi:10.1097/PSY.0b013e318c19a

Buettner, D. (2012, October 24). The enchanted island of centenarians. *The New York Times Magazine.* Available at http://www.nytimes.com/2012/10/28/magazine/the-island-where-people-forget-to-die.html?pagewanted=2&_r=0&hp

Burns, D. (1980). *The feeling good handbook.* New York, NY: Plume.

Caprariello, P. A., & Reis, H. T. (2013). To do, to have, or to share? Valuing experiences over material possessions depends on the involvement of others. *Journal of Personality and Social Psychology, 104,* 199–215. doi:10.1037/a0030953

Coan, J. A., Schaefer, H. S., & Davidson, R. J. (2005, September). *Spouse, but not stranger, hand holding attenuates activation in neural systems underlying response to threat.* Poster presented at the Society for Psychophysiological Research annual meeting, Lisbon, Portugal.

Csikzentmihalyi, M. (2008). *Flow.* New York, NY: Harper Perennial.

Dalai Lama & Cutler, H. C. (2009). *The art of happiness: A handbook for living.* New York, NY: Riverhead Books.

Davis, D., & Hayes, J. (2012, July). What are the benefits of mindfulness? *The Monitor on Psychology, 43*(7), 64.

Diener, E., & Biswas-Diener, R. (2008). *Happiness: Unlocking the mysteries of psychological wealth.* Malden, MA: Blackwell.

Diener, E., & Chan, M. (2010). Happy people live longer: Subjective well-being contributes to health and longevity. *Applied Psychology: Health and Well-Being, 3*(1), 1–43. doi:10.1111/j.1758-0854.2010.01045x

Dolan, Y. M. (1991). *Resolving sexual abuse: Solution-focused therapy and Eriksonian hypnosis for adult survivors.* New York, NY: W. W. Norton & Company.

Doran, G. T. (1981). There's a S.M.A.R.T. way to write management's goals and objectives. *Management Review, 70*(11), 35–36.

Dunn, E. W., Aknin, L. B., & Norton, M. I. (2008). Spending money on others promotes happiness. *Science, 319,* 1687–1688. doi:10.1126/science.1150952

Eaton, N., Keyes, K. M., Krueger, R. F., Balsis, S., Skodol, A. E., Markon, K. E., . . . Hasin, D. S. (2012). An invariant dimensional liability model of gender differences in mental disorder prevalence: Evidence from a national sample. *Journal of Abnormal Psychology, 12*(1), 282–288. doi:10.1037/a0024780

Emmons, R. A., & McCullough, M. E. (2003). Counting blessings versus burdens: An experimental investigation of gratitude and subjective well-being in daily life. *Journal of Personality and Social Psychology, 84,* 377–389. doi:10.1037/0022-3514.84.2.377

Estruch, R. (2013). Primary prevention of cardiovascular disease with a Mediterranean diet. *New England Journal of Medicine, 368,* 1270–1290. Retrieved from http://www.nejm.org/doi/full/10.1056/NEJMoa1200303

Flam, L. (2011, December 6). 91-year-old yoga teacher asks, "Why should I quit?" *NBC News.* Retrieved from http://www.today.com/id/45484875/ns/today-today_health/t/-year-old-yoga-teacher-asks-why-should-i-quit/#.UU4ABBesiSo

Fredrickson, B. (2012). *Positivity: Top-notch research reveals the 3-to-1 ratio that will change your life.* New York, NY: Crown.

Friedman, H., & Martin, L. (2011). *The longevity project.* New York, NY: Hudson Street Press.

Goleman, D. (2006). *Social intelligence.* New York, NY: Bantam Dell.

Goud, N. (2001, October). Sound observations. *Infochange: A publication of the Association for Humanistic Counseling, 100,* 7–9.

Grateful teens are not as likely as their less thankful peers to abuse drugs and alcohol or have behavior problems at school. (2012). *Monitor on Psychology, 43*(9), 12. Retrieved from http://www.apa.org/monitor/2012/10/inbrief.aspx

Haidt, J. (2006). *The happiness hypothesis: Finding modern truths in ancient wisdom.* New York, NY: Basic Books.

Hayes, S. (2008, October). *Acceptance and commitment therapy* [DVD]. Washington, DC: American Psychological Association. (Available from the American Psychological Association, http://www.apa.org/pubs/videos)

Jayson, S. (2012, January 13–15). Stress. *USA Weekend.*

Kabat-Zinn, J. (1994). *Wherever you go, there you are.* New York, NY: Hyperion Press.

King, K. B., & Reis, H. T. (2012). Marriage and long-term survival after coronary artery bypass grafting. *Health Psychology, 31,* 55–62. doi:10.1037/a0025061

Leary, M. R., Tate, E. B., Adams, C. E., Allen, A. B., & Hancock, J. (2007). Self-compassion and reactions to unpleasant self-relevant events: The implications of treating oneself kindly. *Journal of Personality and Social Psychology, 92,* 887–904. doi:10.1037/0022-3514.92.5.887

Lerner, J. S., & Sherman, G. D. (2012, October 29). Gray matter: It isn't easy being king. *The New York Times,* p. 14.

Linley, A., Willars, J., & Biswas-Diener, R. (2010). *The strengths book.* Coventry, England: CAPP Press.

Love helps keep the heart pumping. (2011). *Monitor on Psychology, 42*(10), 16. Retrieved from http://www.apa.org/monitor/2011/11/inbrief.aspx

Love, P., & Carlson, J. (2011). *Never be lonely again: The way out of emptiness, isolation, and a life unfulfilled* (p. 99). Deerfield Park, FL: Health Communications.

Lowndes, L. (2003). *How to talk to anyone.* New York, NY: McGraw-Hill.

Lyubomirsky, S. (2007). *The how of happiness: A scientific approach to getting the life you want.* New York, NY: Penguin Press.

Mann, T., Tomiyama, A. J., Westling, E., Lew, M., Samuels, B., & Chatman, J. (2007). Medicare's search for obesity treatments: Diets are not the answer. *American Psychologist, 62,* 220–233. doi:10.1037/0003-066X.62.3.220

Mayo Clinic. (2013). *Seasonal affective disorder treatment: Choosing a light box.* Retrieved from http://www.mayoclinic.com/health/seasonal-affective-disorder-treatment/DN00013

Medina, J. (2008). *Brain rules.* Seattle, WA: Pear Press.

Medline, National Institutes of Health. (2013). *Autoimmune diseases.* Retrieved from http://www.nlm.nih.gov/medlineplus/autoimmunediseases.html

Muraven, M., Baumeister, R. F., & Tice, D. M. (1999). Longitudinal improvement of self-regulation through practice: Building self-control strength through repeated exercise. *Journal of Social Psychology, 139,* 446–457. doi:10.1080/00224549909598404

Neff, K. (2011). *Self-compassion: Stop beating yourself up and leave insecurity behind.* New York, NY: William Morrow.

Nhat Hanh, T. (1976). *The Miracle of mindfulness: An introduction to the practice of meditation.* Boston, MA: Beacon Press.

Nhat Hanh, T. (1992). *Touching peace: Practicing the art of mindful living.* Berkeley, CA: Parallax Press.

Nhat Hanh, T., & Cheung, L. (2010). *Mindful eating.* New York, NY: HarperOne.

Norcross, J. C., Mrykalo, M. S., & Blagys, M. D. (2002). Auld Lang Syne: Success predictors, change processes, and self-reported outcomes of

New Year's resolvers and nonresolvers. *Journal of Clinical Psychology, 58*, 397–405. doi:10.1002/jclp.1151

Roenneberg, T., Allebrandt, K. V., Merrow, M., & Vetter, C. (2012). Social jetlag and obesity. *Current Biology, 22*, 939–943. doi:10.1016/j.cub.2012.03.038

Sapolsky, R. (2004). *Why zebras don't get ulcers* (3rd ed.). New York, NY: Henry Holt.

Seligman, M. (2011). *Flourish: A visionary new understanding of happiness and well-being.* New York, NY: Free Press.

Shelley E. Taylor. (2010). *Social Psychology Network.* Retrieved from http://shelley.taylor.socialpsychology.org/

Siegel, R. D., Urdang, M. H., & Johnson, D. R. (2001). *Back sense: A revolutionary approach to halting the cycle of chronic back pain.* New York, NY: Broadway Books.

Simon, R. (Ed.). (2011, September/October). Do we even need any psychotherapy anymore? [Special issue]. *Psychotherapy Networker.*

Smits, J., & Otto, M. (2011). *Exercise for mood and anxiety: Proven strategies for overcoming depression and enhancing well-being.* New York, NY: Oxford University Press.

Sterling, T., & Furtula, A. (2011, May 22). Wim Hof, Dutch "iceman," controls body through meditation. *Huffington Post.* Retrieved from http://www.huffingtonpost.com/2011/05/22/wim-hof-dutch-iceman-cont_n_865203.html

Sudsuang, R., Chentanez, V., & Veluvan, K. (1991). Effects of Buddhist meditation on serum cortisol and total protein levels, blood pressure, pulse rate, lung volume and reaction time. *Physiological Behavior, 50*, 543–548.

Walsh, R. (2011). Lifestyle and mental health. *American Psychologist, 66*, 579–592. doi:10.1037/a0021769

Wansink, B., Painter, J. E., & North, J. (2005). Bottomless bowls: Why visual cues of portion size may influence intake. *Obesity Research, 13* 93–100.

Wegner, D. M. (2011). Setting free the bears: Escape from thought suppression. *American Psychologist, 66*, 671–680. doi:10.1037/a0024985

Weir, K. (2011). The exercise effect. *Monitor on Psychology, 42*(11), 49–52.

Weir, K. (2012). The power of self-control. *Monitor on Psychology, 43*(1), 36–38.

Winerman, L. (2011, October). How to eat better—mindlessly. *Monitor on Psychology, 42*(9), 46–47.

Wylie, M. S. (2008, March/April). Sleepless in America: Making it through the night in a wired world. *Psychotherapy Networker.* Retrieved from http://www.psychotherapynetworker.org/magazine/populartopics/140-sleepless-in-america

Younger, J., Aron, A., Parke, S., Chatterjee, N., Mackey, S. (2010). Viewing pictures of a romantic partner reduces experimental pain: Involvement of neural reward systems. *PLoS ONE, 5*(10): e13309. doi:10.1371/journal.pone.0013309

INDEX

ABOUT THE AUTHOR

Pamela A. Hays, PhD, is the author of *Addressing Cultural Complexities in Practice: Assessment, Diagnosis, and Therapy,* and *Connecting Across Cultures: The Helper's Toolkit,* as well as coeditor of *Culturally Responsive Cognitive–Behavioral Therapy.* She holds a doctorate in clinical psychology from the University of Hawaii and from 1987 to 1988 served as a National Institute of Mental Health postdoctoral fellow at the University of Rochester School of Medicine. From 1989 to 2000, she worked as a core faculty member of the graduate psychology program at Antioch University Seattle, where she continues to teach once a year as adjunct. Dr. Hays's research has included work with Vietnamese, Lao, and Cambodian people living in the United States and with Arab Muslim women living in North Africa. Since 2000, she has been back in her hometown of Soldotna, Alaska, working in private practice and as a supervisor for the Kenaitze Tribe's Nakenu Family Center in Kenai, Alaska. She conducts workshops internationally and can be reached at http://www.drpamelahays.com.